THE ESSENTIAL GUIDE TO

COSMETIC LASER SURGERY

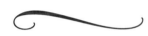

The Revolutionary New Way to
Erase Wrinkles, Age Spots, Scars,
Birthmarks, Moles, Tattoos

...and how not to get burned in the process

BY
Tina Alster, M.D. and Lydia Preston

D1632208

ALLIANCE PUBLISHERS

ISBN 1-887110-09-7

Cover design by Cynthia Dunne
Interior design by Neuwirth & Associates

Alliance books are available at special discounts for bulk purchases for
sales and promotions, premiums, fund raising, or educational use.
Authors are available for public appearances and interviews.
For details, contact:
Alliance Publishing. Inc.
P.O. Box 080377
Brooklyn, New York 11208-0002

Distributed to the trade by National Book Network, Inc.

10 9 8 7 6 5 4 3 2 1

Dedication

To our husbands, Paul Frazer and Jim Hicks, and to our children, Nicholas Alexander Frazer, William Preston Hicks and Blair Montgomery Hicks, with gratitude for their support and forbearance during the writing of this book.

And to the staff of the Washington Institute of Dermatologic Laser Surgery and the patients who so generously shared their experiences and insights.

CONTENTS

FOREWORD

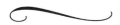

BY

TINA ALSTER, M.D.

Most of us have something or other on our skin we would just as soon be without—a mole, a pock-mark or a crop of freckles. Some people feel self-conscious about little red spots or networks of tiny spider veins. Others regret an impulsively acquired tattoo, or live with prominent scars from surgery or a painful injury. Many people are burdened with birthmarks. And, of course, everyone eventually gets wrinkles—inexorably acquiring the tracery of fine lines and ever deepening furrows that tell of advancing age.

Until very recently, almost all of these marks, from the least noticeable to the grossly disfiguring, had one thing in common. They were virtually impossible to remove without creating some other kind of mark—a scar, a change in skin texture or a patch of unnatural color. Dermatologic cosmetic lasers—a group of highly specialized surgical tools developed in the past decade—have changed that.

These extraordinary new medical instruments have

revolutionized the practice of dermatology, leading to innovative treatments for a host of skin conditions that only a few years ago were regarded as all but intractable. Today there are lasers that can smooth a complexion pitted by acne or chickenpox. Others can remove spider veins, cherry spots, age spots or café-au-lait birthmarks. We can now erase tattoos or restore burned or scarred skin to a more normal appearance. Unsightly moles that once could only be cut out with a scalpel are now vaporized in a burst of laser light. And in one of the closest things we have to a true miracle in medical technology, there is now a laser that eradicates port-wine stains—the dark purplish blotches recognized through the centuries as among the most emotionally ravaging of common birth defects.

Recently, new high-energy carbon dioxide lasers that literally evaporate skin cells have become the most feverishly hyped weapons in the war on wrinkles. Commercially introduced in 1994, the first "UltraPulse" laser received so much media attention for its capacity to bloodlessly peel away lined, age-mottled skin, that thousands of new patients crowded into the offices of doctors employing it. On the horizon are laser treatments that one day may erase stretch marks, permanently remove unwanted hair, eliminate psoriasis and excise dangerous skin cancers with minimal complications.

This frontier has expanded with breathtaking speed. Medical lasers have been in existence for more than thirty years. But until very recently their use in dermatology was limited to a few innovative physicians and university research facilities. My interest was sparked in the 1980s during my residency at Yale University when a woman with a disfiguring port-wine stain consulted me regarding its removal. My search for a treatment for that patient led me to a laser surgery fellowship at Harvard, where I was privileged to join the doctors conducting early clinical trials of the revolutionary new laser invented to treat those stigmatizing birthmarks. When I opened my Washington, DC practice in 1990, I was one of only a handful of board-certified dermatologists or cosmetic surgeons in the United States who owned dermatologic lasers and used them on a regular basis. For the most part, my patients had heard about lasers only through word-of-mouth.

Today thousands of physicians have added cosmetic lasers to their practices. Countless studies on laser use are underway in universities, hospitals and clinical settings. And lately it seems that hardly a week goes by without a magazine article or television news story on the miracles of dermatologic lasers.

These days most of my patients come to me having heard quite a bit about lasers. Unfortunately much of what they have heard is misleading. Lasers are not magic wands. They will not replace a face-lift or give you the flawless complexion of an infant. They cannot cure every unsightly or pathological skin condition. And while laser surgery is, on the whole, less painful and risky than many of the techniques it has replaced, it is still surgery, with the potential complications that attend any surgical procedure.

Is it an option for you?

This book is written to help you make that decision. It is not intended to be a substitute for medical advice. Laser treatment, like any other medical procedure, is something you must discuss with your own physician. This book should help you make the most of that discussion.

It will tell you how different lasers work and how they are employed on a variety of skin conditions. It will give you guidelines on how to find a qualified laser surgeon and how to talk with him or her about possible treatments. It will explain what to anticipate in terms of risk, pain, recovery time and expense. And above all, it will give you an idea of what you can realistically expect to gain—whether your goal is to rid yourself of the burden of a significant disfigurement or to gently erase the marks of the passing years.

INTRODUCTION

How I First Encountered Cosmetic Lasers
BY
Lydia Preston

*T*he first time I walked into Dr. Tina Alster's office I was chagrined to see my bright red face in the mirror I passed on my way through the door. It was a bitter December afternoon and the cold air outside had brought out the mottled scarlet flush across my cheeks, nose and chin that is typical of rosacea—a skin condition characterized by chronically dilated capillaries in the face.

"I look like Rudolf the Red-Nosed Reindeer," I exclaimed in despair. The doctor, a petite blonde with an enviable porcelain complexion and the upbeat manner of the varsity cheerleader she once was, laughed sympathetically. Then she said, to my astonishment, "We can certainly fix *that* for you."

Until that moment, I hadn't a clue that there was any kind of a treatment at all for my red cheeks and nose. I had been told that they were permanent—like W.C. Fields' bulbous red "drinker's nose," which is a side effect of rosacea in advanced stages. I had come to see Dr. Alster for another problem. A couple of weeks earlier I had read a magazine article about a new wrinkle-removing laser. The story mentioned in passing that some physicians were using the same laser experimentally on acne scars. I wanted to know if there was anything that could be done for the dozen or so distinct scars that marked my cheeks—visible reminders of adolescent breakouts that had stubbornly persisted into my thirties.

Neither the acne scars nor the rosacea could be called disfiguring. But I was self-conscious about both. My face usually looked ruddy and rough textured. And the embarrassing fluorescent red could flare up in an instant with exertion, sudden changes in temperature, a hot drink or a spicy meal—things I had been told to avoid in order to control the flushing. A plastic surgeon with whom I had consulted had advised against treating the acne scars with dermabrasion or a chemical peel, both of which carry some risk of scarring or permanent pigment changes. "Your skin really isn't that bad," he consoled. "You can always cover it with makeup." Of course, I had been doing that scrupulously for more than 30 years, ever since my face started breaking out when I was a teenager.

Six months after my first consultation with Dr. Alster, I shifted my bottles of foundation to the back of the medicine cabinet. After two laser treatments—one to remove the network of dilated blood vessels, the other to smooth out the acne scars—I now go for days without using any makeup at all, greeting the world with nothing on my face but sunscreen.

My skin is not perfect. I still flush easily and remain sensitive to extremes in temperature. And the acne scars, while much reduced, can still be detected under close inspection. But for the first time in my adult life the skin on my face generally appears clear, smooth and normal. For me, that counts as a medical miracle.

It is, of course, a minor miracle compared to those that have occurred in the lives of the many people whose far more serious skin disorders have been successfully treated with dermatologic lasers since these specialized instruments came of age in the late 1980s. Since my own first encounters with laser surgery, I've spoken to dozens of Dr. Alster's other patients and watched as she's operated on many of them. I have met men and women whose lives have been transformed and children whose personalities have blossomed after being freed of disfiguring birthmarks or the devastating scars left by burns, accidents or serious surgery. I've seen people jubilant over finally getting rid of an embarrassing tattoo, a prominent mole, or some other unsightly skin feature that's been eroding their self-confidence for years. And I've watched a steady stream of individuals in their 40s, 50s, 60s, even older—men as well as women—as they have had a decade or more wiped from their faces along with their crow's feet, lip wrinkles or liver spots.

Seeing these patients and hearing their stories—many of which are recounted in the following pages—it sometimes seems that cosmetic lasers do indeed have magical properties. But, as anyone who may be contemplating laser surgery should know, they do not. Lasers are sophisticated medical tools that perform certain specific procedures in a uniquely effective manner. And they demonstrate exceptional potential for the future.

However, the intense publicity that lasers have received in recent years has created extraordinary, often unrealistic expectations. Sometimes the results of laser surgery are modest and subtle, disappointing those who have been led to expect the miraculous. And at other times this new, rapidly developing technology is used inappropriately—with disastrous consequences. Remember, lasers can cut steel. They can certainly do some terrible damage to your skin. So it behooves you to be both cautious and highly skeptical when investigating laser surgery for yourself. Here are a few things that any potential consumer of laser surgery should bear in mind:

▶ Most dermatologic laser procedures are highly technique-dependent. This means that the results are directly proportional to the skill and experience of the surgeon. "There are so many variables you have to bear in mind and so many ways you can go wrong," says Dr. Alster, who in the past few years has seen her caseload increase with a small but alarming new class of patients: those coming to her to treat serious scars left by less experienced laser practitioners.

▶ Laser surgery is a completely unregulated specialty and most physicians now practicing it are essentially learning on the job. There is nothing to stop anyone with an MD or a degree in osteopathic medicine from buying a laser and aiming it at patients that very day—with no more training than whatever instructions they receive from the manufacturer's sales representative. Reputable physicians do not behave so recklessly. But even those who carefully study this rapidly evolving new specialty and proceed to practice it cautiously can take many months to acquire the skills that are needed to safely and effectively achieve the best results.

▶ Dermatologic lasers are not all-purpose tools. Each of those in current clinical use is a highly specialized instrument specifically designed to treat a carefully defined class of related skin conditions. Some of the worst mistakes come from using inappropriate or outdated machines.

► Finally, lasers are expensive. "When I moved to Washington, I bought my first lasers instead of a house," says Dr. Alster. The dermatologic lasers in most common use today cost from $95,000 to $120,000 each. And they require average annual maintenance fees amounting to some $5,000 to $20,000 apiece. A well-equipped practice needs a minimum of four lasers—and should be prepared to replace them as the technology improves. This, of course, represents a substantial investment for any private practitioner and it has two obvious direct effects on consumers. First of all, the lasers' costs are reflected in very high fees— fees that for the most part are not covered by medical insurance. And second, physicians who have invested close to half a million dollars in lasers have tremendous incentive to make their new equipment pay—prompting some of them to encourage laser surgery for conditions that might be treated just as effectively and more cheaply by other means.

The bottom line is this: Without giving considerable thought to whether or not you are a suitable candidate for laser surgery and without taking real care in selecting a doctor, you can wind up paying a lot of money for a very disappointing, even devastating outcome. We hope that this book, which combines Dr. Alster's expertise with my own perspective as a patient and a reporter, and with the insights and experiences of hundreds of her other patients, will help you avoid that.

The word **laser** is an acronym. It stands for **L**ight **A**mplification by **S**timulated **E**mission of **R**adiation. Simply speaking, a laser is a device that emits a special kind of light. The light creates energy inside a chamber, where it is amplified into a highly focused, extremely intense beam—powerful enough to facet a diamond. Dermatologists and cosmetic surgeons have been experimenting with this technology since the 1960s, when physicians first began using laser beams like space-age scalpels in specialties such as ophthalmology. But the first dermatologic lasers often produced disastrous burns and, for the most part, were hastily dropped from the medical arsenal.

Today's cosmetic lasers are not cutting tools, but sophisticated search and destroy weapons. They were developed according to a principle known as **selective photothermolysis**. Essentially, this means that you can adjust a laser beam so that it destroys a specific organic target. By passing the light through different dyes, crystals or gasses, you can manipulate its color and wavelength so that it zeroes in on the targeted molecules without damaging surrounding tissues.

This is the basis for the innovative flashlamp-pumped pulsed dye laser that revolutionized the treatment of port-wine birthmarks. The yellow beam of light that is produced by the dye-containing laser chamber is tuned to the hemoglobin in red blood cells. The light passes harmlessly through the skin's surface as if through a pane of glass, enters a blood vessel and hits the red cells. As they absorb the light energy, the cells instantly heat up and the blood in that area boils like hot water in a pipe, destroying the vessel walls. Working on one pencil eraser-sized spot at a time, a laser surgeon can thus methodically eliminate the collection of abnormal blood vessels that constitute a port-wine stain, leaving the overlying skin smooth and unscarred.

Other dermatologic lasers, designed to treat other skin problems, emit light tuned to different targets—the water in surface skin cells, for example, or the ink particles that make up a tattoo. In most of these lasers, the beam is pulsed, which means that the light fires on and off in extremely short bursts. The pulses, much too rapid for the human eye to see, ensure that heat generated by the laser does not build up in the targeted area so that it spreads by conduction to nearby skin cells—the damaging effect produced by the older, so-called continuous wave lasers that so frequently were responsible for burning or scarring patients.

CHAPTER ONE

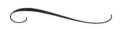

A New Way to a New Face

*I*n the laser room, Alix reclined in a big adjustable chair like those in a dentist's office. Her face had been scrubbed bare of makeup, and her eyes were covered with tiny opaque plastic goggles. Under the bright surgical lights, the signs of age that 52 years had etched into her skin stood out in clear relief. Crows' feet radiated out from the corners of her eyes and vertical frown lines cut between her brows. Horizontal grooves creased her forehead and deep furrows ran from the sides of her nose to the corners of her mouth. A starburst of wrinkles puckered her lips.

As with everyone her age, the passage of years, heredity, and the good and bad habits of a lifetime had combined their effects to give Alix her face at mid-life. The damage left by long summers in the sun was apparent all over her skin—in its coarse texture and network of lines, in scattered brown splotches and small scaly patches. The broad, somewhat heavy eyelids she had inherited from her mother—a distinctive and attractive

TINA ALSTER, M.D. & LYDIA PRESTON

feature of her youth—had drooped with age, giving her blue eyes a tired, hooded look. The pull of gravity was equally apparent in the soft, loose skin under her chin and along her jawline. Even her outgoing personality had taken a toll, her natural vivacity acting to deepen the expression lines of her characteristically animated face.

Alix had kept her body in shape, so from a distance, she did not appear much different from her two teenage daughters. But up close, she looked her age. In fact, like many healthy and active women in their 40s or 50s, she thought she actually looked a lot older than her age—certainly far older than she felt.

"I was thinking about getting a face lift. I spent a lot of time in front of the mirror, pulling the skin back under my neck and around the eyes, just to see what would happen."

What happened was that even a small amount of stretching seemed to subtly alter her features. And when she pulled her skin hard enough to smooth out the wrinkles, she looked as if she were trapped in a wind tunnel.

"I was afraid of a face lift. I thought it would change me too much. And anyway, no matter how hard I tugged, it didn't do anything to the lines around my mouth."

Laser surgery offered Alix an alternative—a way to smooth out the wrinkles and rejuvenate her skin without radically changing her basic appearance as she feared a face lift might. So she decided to take the plunge, and here she was, ready to undergo a full-face resurfacing procedure that would bloodlessly remove the corrugated, sun-damaged upper layers of skin and make her face a clean slate.

With her eyes covered, and heavily sedated to ease the pain of the procedure, Alix was almost completely unaware of what was happening. It took less than an hour, and about 45 minutes after that, still a little shaky from the anesthesia, she was sent home.

Her face, coated with protective ointment, was red, raw and starting to swell. By the next morning, it had ballooned up to the size of a basketball. "It was so painful even my teeth hurt."

Over the next few days—with her eyes swollen nearly shut and her laser-treated skin oozing and crusting—Alix thought she must have been insane to do such a thing to herself. But by the end of the week, the swelling had subsided and a new layer of surface skin cells had built up. Her face was still tender. And it was still bright red. But she had begun to look more like her normal self.

Three weeks later, Alix celebrated Thanksgiving with a dramatically different face—younger and healthier looking than it had appeared in over a decade. Her skin was still distinctly red, but the color was uniform, minus the splotches and irregular brownish spots.

And it was miraculously smooth. The fine lines that had made her cheeks and chin look like crumpled tissue paper were gone, along with the sharp little puckers around her mouth and the deep hash marks that had slashed from her lower lip down her chin. The skin under her eyes had tightened and lost its lax, crepe-like texture. Even her hooded lids had lifted.

Six months after her operation, the point where laser resurfacing patients are considered substantially healed and able to see what their long-term results will be, Alix noticed that a few lines had returned. The creases across her forehead, between her brows and from her nose to her mouth—all attached to facial muscles she used every day to smile, laugh or frown—were back. But they were softer, shallower and less harshly aging than before. And they would remain that way for long into the future.

As for all of the other wrinkles, they were gone for good.

New ones would gradually appear over the following years as Alix continued to age normally—for while laser surgery can turn back the clock, it can't stop it. But Alix figured she had bought herself a decade. At least. It was not just what she saw in the mirror, or heard in the voices of friends telling her she looked 10 years younger, that convinced her. It was also what happened when she got a new driver's license. The examiner puzzled over her birthdate, looked at her old photo and finally decided, "Oh, you've lost weight."

"Which I hadn't," Alix recalled. "I'd actually put on a pound or two since the old picture was taken. But my face had tightened up to that extent."

And then there was the conversation with a casual acquaintance, someone around her own age, who said matter-of-factly, "Of course you wouldn't remember the '50s. You weren't around in the '50s."

"I was born in 1943! Of course I remember the '50s. But imagine hearing somebody say something like that. That's when I know I really got something. That it was worth it. Really, really worth it."

LASER MYTHS AND REALITY

Not everyone sees such dramatic improvement in their skin following laser resurfacing. But many people have. And they are living proof that the wrinkle-removing lasers so widely touted in magazines, on TV, and in the advertising of many of the physicians now entering this new field, really can erase years from your face. And they can do it quickly and bloodlessly, restoring an old, lined, rough surface to youthful smoothness without the risks and potentially serious side effects of other forms of cosmetic surgery.

Yet, as Alix's experience also demonstrates, it is neither as simple nor as easy as it is sometimes made out to be. Laser resurfacing, or laserbrasion as it is also called, is still essentially in its infancy as a surgical procedure, and misconceptions about it abound.

It is not at all unusual to read accounts in the popular press that promise a virtually pain-free experience and blithely predict "about a week" of recovery time. The truth is that while laser resurfacing does not involve the incisions, stitches and bruising of conventional cosmetic procedures, it is still traumatic and painful. Resurfacing removes the top layers of the skin, which is a tremendous insult to the human body. And although it takes only a week or so for the body to rebuild its missing surface, this represents only the first stage of healing. Complete recovery can take up to a year.

Most patients—and some doctors who are new to lasers—are surprised at how much time is involved. Even people who have been thoroughly briefed in advance often express shock at the initial pain, the prolonged period of skin redness that follows, and the number of follow-up visits that are needed. "Grueling" is a word often used to describe the process by those who have gone through it.

"People watch those stories on TV and they think it's nothing. Boy, are they in for a surprise," said Louise, a 46-year-old attorney who had laser resurfacing surgery on a Thursday afternoon in Washington, DC, and that evening, against medical advice, flew to Texas for the weekend. She wound up in a Dallas emergency room, in terrible pain, and looking "Gross, like a big red balloon. Nobody knew what had happened to me. And nobody knew what to do for me."

"My eyes were swollen completely shut," recalled Danielle, who had laserbrasion around her eyes, where at the age of 39, she had detected her first wrinkles. "It was horrible."

"I cried for five days," added Terry, also 39. "I kept saying why did I do this? Why did I do this?"

THE REASONS WHY

The answers to why people undergo any form of cosmetic surgery are highly personal and individual. They are rooted in an apparently universal human desire to appear as attractive and as healthy as possible. And in a culture that puts a premium on youth, looking attractive and healthy is equated with looking young—or at least younger.

People frequently point out that this is particularly true in the contemporary job market. As one woman bluntly put it, "It's a competitive world. When you look young, you've got an edge. When you start to look old, you lose it."

Other patients have other concerns. Roberta, widowed in her mid-40s, said she felt that grief at her husband's death was written in every line on her face. "My eyes drooped. My mouth drooped. Just looking so sad and depressed made everything seem worse." Laser surgery two years later "helped me feel like I could move on. It seems so superficial. But when I started to look better, I began to feel better."

And again and again, patients say they find it disconcerting to look so much older than they feel. It's a common complaint, rooted in a simple fact about aging. Most people do look older than their years because up to 90 percent of the visible signs of age derive from damage caused by overexposure to the sun. Photo-aging, as it is called, puts many more wrinkles in people's faces than chronological aging or "just getting old." Erasing sun damage—the laser's forte—usually makes people's faces look as their biological destiny intended. Most patients find that to be just about the right degree of improvement in their appearance.

"I'm not a girl and I don't want to look like one. But all those wrinkles and age spots on my face made me look so tired and worn out all the time," explained Alix. "People say I look so much younger than my age now. I really don't think that's true. I think I look just about like any woman my age should."

Of course there are others who frankly *do* want to look younger than their age. "I never want to look any older than I do right now," cheerfully confessed Danielle, vowing to "do anything it takes" to keep the signs of age at bay.

For all of these patients and many others laser surgery offers an accessible middle ground between watching their wrinkles deepen and making the often dramatic corrections of conventional plastic surgery—-a step many people are not willing to take for a number of reasons.

Danielle felt she was still too young for the face lift she still intends to have in her 40s. "I think this will hold me until then," she said.

Others are frankly scared of conventional surgery. "I don't want anyone cutting my face," stated one woman emphatically. Many are concerned, as Alix was, that a face lift may change their appearance too radically, making them look artificially young.

"This is more subtle," said Louise, comparing the final results of her laser surgery with the eye lift she had four years earlier. "But I think I look gorgeous. I lost all my wrinkles, all my sun damage. Clients tell me I look younger. I'd do it again. In fact I probably will do it again. "

"When the swelling went down, it looked amazing," said Terry. "I'd do it again in a heartbeat."

Alix agreed: "It was difficult, yes. But I'd definitely do it again."

Laser resurfacing cannot replace a surgical lift, which works in an entirely different way to attack wrinkles. Face lifts, brow lifts and eye lifts (blepharoplasty) all tighten the skin by literally lifting it up and pulling it over the underlying facial bones. Excess skin is cut away and deep creases are stretched smooth; frequently underlying musculature is surgically rearranged. This is the only way to correct the slackness, sagging and heavy folds that occur around the neck, jowls and eyes as a person ages.

But face lifts have only a moderately smoothing effect on superficial wrinkles and on "expression lines"—the furrows carved between the eyes by repeatedly knitting your brows, the folds from nose to mouth that deepen when you smile, the squint lines and crows' feet that crinkle the outer corners of your eyes, or the little "lipstick bleed" lines that pucker your lips. These wrinkles may become less noticeable in the newly taut surface after a face lift. However, a surgeon who pulls the skin too hard in an effort to get rid of every surface flaw can produce an abnormally tight, distorted look—the weird eagle eyes or the widely stretched mouth that screams "Bad Face Lift!"

Expression lines, or dynamic wrinkles as they are called, are often more successfully treated with various line filling agents—substances that are injected or implanted beneath the skin to fill out the depressions. The most common line fillers are collagen, autologous fat—that is, fat cells harvested from elsewhere in the patient's body—and Fibrel, a gel-like material that is mixed into a paste with the patient's own blood. (Liquid silicone, once widely employed to plump up wrinkles, is no longer used for that purpose in the United States because of the serious complications it sometimes produced.)

Another type of wrinkle-fighting injection involves the use of botulism toxin, or "Botox." Developed by the military as a chemical weapon, Botox is a potent neurotoxin. Injected into frown lines in extremely tiny doses, it paralyzes the muscles that cause the lines—relaxing them into smoothness.

Wrinkle-fighting injections are popular with many patients because they are relatively inexpensive and offer quick results. In the case of collagen, you can get your lines filled out in the morning and sail off to a party that night. But none of the line fillers last very long. The body immediately starts to absorb the injected material and the shots must be repeated every few months to maintain the effect. Botox wears off quickly too— usually in about three to five months—although with time, the muscles responsible for the lines become smaller through lack of use, permanently softening the affected areas.

Risks, magnified by the need for repeat injections, include scarring from the needles, infection and allergic reactions. Another possible side effect is fibrosis—a condition character- ized by areas of tough, abnormally thickened, scar-like tissue that form under the treated skin in response to the foreign agent. Botox carries the additional risk of accidentally paralyz- ing small muscles close to the eyes, causing the lids to droop shut.

Neither face lifts nor injections remove fine, superficial wrinkles on the cheeks and chin or around the eyes. These wrinkles are largely due to sun damage. Over the years, ultra- violet rays penetrate the upper layer of the unprotected epider- mis, progressively damaging the fibrous collagen support structure that lies in the dermis just below. Gradually this lat- ticework of supportive material breaks down and the surface crumples into dozens of wrinkles called solar rhytides.

Two skin resurfacing methods, dermabrasion and chemical peels, are the traditional means of smoothing out solar rhytides and improving the surface texture of the skin. They are also often used to remove other types of superficial damage, including the flat brown spots or liver spots (solar lentigines, as doctors call them) that give aging skin its mottled look, or the irregular, scaly, reddish growths (actinic keratoses), that are the precursors to certain kinds of skin cancers.

With dermabrasion, a rapidly rotating, abrasive metal wheel is used like a carpenter's sander to mechanically scrape off the skin's surface. It is a gory procedure. Blood wells up instantly on the skin. The air fills with a red mist from droplets spraying off the wheel and the operating room takes on the atmosphere of an abattoir. "It was just awful," recalled Emily, 41, of the dermabrasion she had for acne scarring in her 30s. "The blood sprayed everywhere. I mean, you just can't imagine. And in the end, I wound up with a lot of uneven ridges on my face that I didn't have before."

Indeed, it is extremely difficult for the surgeon to determine how the treatment is progressing and how deeply the skin has been abraded. And often, the end result is a wavy, unnaturally contoured surface, much like an unevenly sanded piece of wood.

Deep chemical peels, in which a caustic acid is applied to the skin to burn off its top layers and the wrinkles they contain, are similarly hard to control. Because of the many subtle and not always obvious variations in people's skin, patients respond differently and unpredictably to chemical peeling agents. Determining how strong a solution to use and calculating how long it should stay on is pretty much a matter of educated guesswork bolstered by intuition.

The safety and effectiveness of both dermabrasion and chemical peels depend on the experience and skill of the surgeon performing them. Both carry considerable risk, even in the most deft hands. Very deep chemical peels using the acid phenol are particularly dangerous because the phenol is absorbed through the skin and taken into the bloodstream like a toxic drug. In some individuals this can cause kidney damage, heart irregularities or other serious medical complications. A few people have actually died as a result of complications from phenol peels.

With either dermabrasion or a chemical peel, it is virtually impossible to predict how the finished surface will look, and the dangers of scarring from abrading or peeling too deeply are considerable. Long-lasting or even permanent color changes are common if the melanocytes—the cells that produce the skin pigment melanin—are damaged. Sometimes the skin turns considerably lighter. Patients who have had a chemical peel or dermabrasion above the lip often wind up with what looks like a milk mustache. Others develop dark brown mottling because their skin reacts to the insult of the procedure by over-producing melanin.

WHAT THE LASER DOES

Just as the term implies, laser resurfacing is simply a new way to resurface skin—essentially an alternative to dermabrasion or chemical peels. Performed correctly, it eliminates or dramatically reduces the risks associated with either of those other techniques, and on the whole, side effects are less serious and more predictable.

Laser resurfacing is performed with a carbon dioxide laser, so called because the laser beam passes through a chamber filled with carbon dioxide (CO_2) gas. Invented in the early

1960s, the CO_2 laser is one of the most powerful tools of modern industry, capable of slicing through two-inch thick steel like a knife through butter. It is a versatile surgical instrument as well, prized for its capacity to cleanly and precisely vaporize tissue. It works on skin by emitting a wavelength that is absorbed by water, the main component of skin cells. The beam heats, boils and instantly evaporates water inside the cells, thus vaporizing the cells in a puff of steam.

The Coherent UltraPulse laser, commercially introduced in 1994, turned this industrial and medical workhorse into a specialized tool for resurfacing skin.. The UltraPulse—which has since inspired similar commercial rivals—electronically breaks the powerful laser beam into extremely short pulses, precisely calibrated to allow heat to dissipate in between. Firing in millisecond bursts, the laser vaporizes skin cells, which literally vanish into thin air before the heat in them travels to adjacent tissues.

When "lasing," as the process is called, a surgeon works on one small area at a time, methodically vaporizing aged, sun-damaged skin, one microscopic layer after another. The procedure is virtually bloodless and does not initially cause swelling, so that the doctor can control precisely how much skin is removed.

As the body heals, it replaces the treated areas with a new, unblemished and significantly smoother surface. Solar rhytides and other sun-induced damage seem wiped away. Fine, crepey wrinkling around the eyes and pucker lines around the mouth disappear.

Much of this improvement is due to the laser's effect on collagen, the fibrous protein that makes up the skin's built-in support fabric. In a mechanism that is still not entirely understood and that does not occur to the same extent in any other form of cosmetic surgery, collagen fibers visibly contract in response to the laser beam. This actually shrinks the skin over the facial structure.

Patients notice the effect about a week after surgery, when the worst of the swelling has gone down. Their skin feels uncomfortably taut. And it looks tighter than it did before, actually mimicking the effects of a face lift in some people.

This extreme tightness—apparently due to the direct effect of heat on the collagen—only lasts a few months. The skin, which continually rebuilds and replenishes itself from the inside out, gradually replaces the affected fibers with new collagen. However, many patients find that their skin continues to feel noticeably tighter than it did before, leading researchers to believe that the laser beam may have a long-term effect on the skin's collagen-producing mechanism. Although no one understands exactly how or why it happens, laboratory examination has shown that the collagen fibers in laser-treated skin are generally more abundant and more regular in shape—in other words, more like "young" collagen—than in skin that has not been treated with the laser.

The phenomenon of collagen remodeling following laser surgery has changed the way some physicians approach other cosmetic surgical procedures. In the past, doctors frequently followed a face, brow or eye lift with chemical resurfacing or dermabrasion to get rid of the fine wrinkles left behind. Today, surgeons increasingly are inclined to use a laser on the superficial wrinkles first, wait several months to see how much the skin tightens as a result, then proceed with the surgical lift.

Sometimes patients who have had laser resurfacing in anticipation of a face lift reconsider afterwards. Connie, who at 45 intended to tighten her baggy eyelids and slackening jaw with blepharoplasty and a "mini-lift" of the chin, changed her mind after laserbrasion. "I'll probably still get a face lift someday. But now I don't think I'll need it until I'm in my 50s." Rosemary, 68, canceled a scheduled face lift after laser surgery on the frown lines between her eyes and the wrinkled skin around her mouth. "It seemed like that's where I saw most of my age, and now that those parts look better, I don't think a face lift would do that much more for me."

"I had no idea that my skin would tighten so much," commented Alix, whose hooded eyelids lifted so noticeably after laser treatment. She also noticed that the slack skin under her jaw seemed to have been pulled up a bit by the all-over tightening of her face—an effect that is hard to measure, but one that other patients have also claimed as a result of full-face laser resurfacing.

As with all other forms of cosmetic surgery, good results depend on experience, judgment and a sensitive hand. The laser must take off enough skin to remove the flaw and create a smooth area to re-epithelialize—that is, to build up a new top layer. But if a surgeon goes too deeply by making too many passes of the beam in one area, he or she will remove too much skin and create a deep injury that the skin cannot repair. The result will be a scar.

The current state of laser technology confines laser resurfacing to the face. The skin there is relatively thick, and boasts an abundance of oil and sweat glands and hair follicles. These small structures—called pilosebaceous units —are lined with epidermal cells that migrate up and out to regenerate the new skin surface. On other parts of the body, such as the neck and chest, or the backs of the hands, the skin is much thinner and has fewer pilosebaceous structures to initiate regrowth of a new surface.

Studies have shown that, on average, skin on the face has

about 30 times as many pilosebaceous units as the skin on the neck and chest; about 40 times as many as the skin on the backs of the hands and arms. This means that those areas always take far longer to heal and are at much greater risk for complications such as infection or scarring. However, lasers can successfully treat isolated lesions on the chest, hands or arms. (See Chapters 4 and 5.)

Other than possible scarring, the most serious potential complication from laser resurfacing surgery is possible pigment change, although, on the whole, skin treated with a laser heals with a more even, normal color than skin subjected to chemical peels or dermabrasion. About 30 percent of patients do experience some temporary degree of hyperpigmentation, or skin darkening. Hypopigmentation, or skin lightening, is possible but rare following laser surgery.

Like dermabrasion or a chemical peel, laser resurfacing cannot totally eradicate every flaw, in particular the wrinkles caused by repetitive facial expressions. These, however, are usually minimized and softened by laser treatment. And, unlike line filling injections, the laser produces permanent results. Whatever the laser beam removes is gone for good—until advancing age or additional sun exposure creates new lines.

Is It a Burn?

The pulsed CO_2 laser used for resurfacing skin generates extremely high temperatures, and patients who have been treated with it look and feel as if they have been badly sunburned. Because of this, people frequently characterize laser resurfacing surgery as a kind of burn. However, the effect on the skin is significantly different.

The laser beam removes the epidermis and part of the dermis—just as a second degree burn does. But the laser's rapidly pulsed action ensures that heat does not build up in underlying tissues or spread out to adjacent areas. Skin untouched by the beam is unharmed and the live, active cells that remain in the skin can work normally to regenerate a new surface. Because the damage inflicted by the laser is uniform, the entire surface heals evenly, at the same pace.

On the other hand, skin that has sustained a true second degree burn—whether from the sun, a flame or some other source—is always affected to a certain extent by heat build-up. Because some sections of skin get hotter than others and are more severely damaged, the surface heals at different rates, in a blotchy, uneven fashion. In addition, the heat has a devastating effect on the remaining skin cells. Sometimes they cannot reproduce normally in order to repair the damage. The result may be light scarring or permanent changes in the collagen, producing a rubbery feeling. Moreover, heat damage may alter the genetic code of the affected cells. The result may only appear years later in the form of squamous cell skin cancers which are seen commonly in skin that has received severe burns.

All skin resurfacing procedures work in essentially the same way—by removing the layers of skin that contain a wrinkle or other flaw, and creating a wound. The wound heals by generating new skin cells that will create a smoother, less flawed surface. The trick lies in removing just enough skin to take out the imperfection without damaging the skin so badly that it cannot repair itself normally. To comprehend just how this is done, it is necessary to understand some basics about how our skin is structured.

Human skin is comprised of three layers. The innermost is the **subcutis** or fatty layer. Above it lies the **dermis**, the skin's fibrous support structure. The dermis consists of a meshwork of protein strands, **collagen** and **elastin**, which actually look very much like the threads that make up woven cloth. Through these fibers run networks of blood vessels and nerves, and so-called **pilosebaceous units**, which are composed of hair follicles connected to sweat glands and oil-producing sebaceous glands.

The dermis is divided into the thick lower, or **reticular dermis**, and the thin upper, or **papillary dermis**, which is composed of tiny projections (papillae) that extend up into the skin's top layer, the **epidermis**. Richly supplied with oxygen and nutrients by capillaries in the papillae, the epidermis constantly produces new cells. Among them are **melanocytes**, which synthesize the skin-darkening pigment **melanin**, and **keratinocytes**, which produce a protein called **keratin**. In a process called keratinization, keratinocytes migrate steadily upward, gradually losing moisture and become stiffer and flatter. They reach the surface as brittle husks, composed entirely of keratin, which form the visible outer layer of the skin, the

stratum corneum, or horny layer.

The effect of any resurfacing technique depends on how deeply a peeling agent penetrates this multi-layered structure. Light salon peels, which involve the application of very low concentrations of glycolic acid, remove the horny layer, which is quickly replaced by a fresh new surface in the ordinary course of cell birth and maturation. Superficial "lunchtime" chemical peels, performed with stronger glycolic solutions, take off the entire epidermis—along with any flaws it might contain. Intact epidermal cells inside the pilosebaceous units generate new cells that travel up the hair follicles to create a new skin surface; other epidermal cells migrate inward from around the edges of the wound.

Light peels improve the skin's surface texture and remove superficial flaws, but they have little effect on wrinkles, which are caused by the breakdown of collagen fibers in the dermis. Wrinkles can be significantly improved only by medium to deep peels employing a strong acid, or by dermabrasion or laserbrasion. Medium depth peels, which typically employ 35% to 50% trichloroacetic acid (TCA) solutions, remove the papillary and upper reticular dermis, which includes the damaged collagen causing the wrinkles. As the skin repairs itself, the dermis' collagen-producing cells (called **fibroblasts**) create new collagen strands that are more regular and abundant than before. The result is a noticeably smoother surface. Deep chemical peels and dermabrasion, which remove tissue all the way down to the mid-reticular dermis, are even more dramatically effective, eliminating shallow wrinkles and significantly smoothing deeper ones.

The mid-reticular dermis is about as far as any resurfacing agent can safely go—removing the upper part of the pilosebaceous units, yet leaving enough of their structure intact to regenerate normal new skin. Peeling any deeper risks destroying the pilosebaceous units, along with the skin's ability to restore itself. Peels that are too deep also damage the pigment-producing melanocytes, which can lead to permanent changes in skin color. And they may destroy or so badly damage the fibroblasts that the skin can no longer produce normal collagen. The resulting development of abnormal collagen fibers creates the scar-like dermal thickening known as tissue fibrosis.

The depth that a laser penetrates depends on how many passes the surgeon makes with the laser beam. Typically, the first pass vaporizes the epidermis, exposing the papillary dermis. Subsequent passes go successively deeper, first vaporizing the loose network of collagen and elastin fibers that comprise the papillary dermis, then progressing steadily deeper into the reticular dermis. The laser's great advantage over other methods is its precision. A skilled surgeon can peel deeply enough to make a significant impact on wrinkles, while stopping just short of compromising the skin's ability to regenerate itself normally. No other resurfacing method reliably affords that degree of control.

CHAPTER TWO

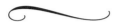

UP IN SMOKE:
HOW WRINKLES ARE VAPORIZED

*L*aserbrasion appears to be simplicity in itself—about as challenging as peeling a piece of fruit. In fact, salesmen for cosmetic laser manufacturers commonly demonstrate their machines by aiming them at fruits and vegetables, stripping the skin off apples, eggplants or tomatoes without bruising or blemishing the flesh beneath. A child could do it.

Lase the skin off a tomato, that is.

But human skin is something entirely different. It is an organ—the body's largest—and it is a complex, living entity. Laser resurfacing removes this crucial organ's protective outer surface, the epidermis. It also removes the top section of the dermis, the skin's fibrous support structure which is full of tiny glands, minute blood vessels and highly sensitive nerve endings that must all be rebuilt. This involves a complex and lengthy healing process.

Three critical factors influence how well the skin heals and determine the results a patient can expect. The first is careful preoperative evaluation and preparation. The second is the skill and experience of the surgeon. And finally, crucially, there is the quality of the follow-up care immediately after the operation and over the ensuing months, both to ensure optimum healing and to arrest any problems that might result in serious complications.

Deciding on Laser Resurfacing

How can you determine if you are a good candidate for laser resurfacing and decide whether or not you really want to go through with it? Here are the key things to consider and discuss with your doctor:

▶ Have realistic expectations. Laser resurfacing smooths the skin and the results are often dramatic. But it's not a face lift. It won't pull up loose, sagging skin; deep expression lines will see only moderate improvement.

▶ Although laser resurfacing has been performed successfully on people over the age of 80, older patients tend to heal more slowly because their skin produces new cells at a slower rate than younger people.

▶ Fair-haired, light-skinned people can generally expect the best, most predictable results. Those with naturally dark or olive skin tones tend to experience prolonged redness after laser surgery and are more likely to show more obvious and longer lasting pigment changes. Because of this, some laser surgeons strongly advise individuals of African or Asian descent not to pursue resurfacing. (See "Dark Skin and Post-Surgical Skin Darkening," pages 48–51.)

► Carefully weigh the pros and cons of having your entire face resurfaced as opposed to concentrating on local areas, such as around the eyes or mouth. It is less costly and somewhat less traumatic to have smaller areas treated. But you will get a more uniform effect from a full-face procedure. Small sections of skin take just as long to heal as larger ones, and for several months—or even longer— there will be a noticeable difference in color between treated areas and the surrounding skin. Over the long term, the lased skin may have a perceptibly smoother texture.

► Tissue fibrosis—underlying thickening of the skin from injuries or previous surgical procedures—alters the manner in which laser light is absorbed. If you have ever had any cosmetic procedure such as dermabrasion, a chemical peel or silicone, collagen or fat injections, those areas may not respond well to the laser beam. Electrolysis to remove hair from the upper lip or the chin sometimes leaves tiny pits or scars that can also interfere with the laser. (CAUTION: Patients sometimes neglect to tell their doctors about previous cosmetic procedures; some even deny having had them. It is essential to inform the surgeon ahead of time so that he or she can adjust the laser accordingly.)

► Choose your time for surgery carefully and plan for a long recovery. You will need a minimum of seven days at home; many people take 10 days off. For several months afterwards your skin will be exceptionally sensitive to the sun. Ideally, you should stay out of sunlight entirely during this period. Many people deliberately schedule laser surgery for fall or winter months when they are less likely to be spending time outdoors.

▶ Moles, red spider veins, warts or any other skin condition should be carefully evaluated by a dermatologist before laser resurfacing. Some skin problems may have to be treated first—perhaps with other laser procedures. If there is any suspicion that a mole or other small growth may be malignant or potentially so, a biopsy may be necessary to rule out cancer before scheduling surgery. Most doctors consider it safe to remove scaly precancerous lesions (actinic keratoses) or superficial basal cell skin cancers in the course of resurfacing with the CO_2 laser (see Chapter 4). In fact, laser resurfacing is now considered one of the best ways to treat mild skin cancers and pre-cancers. However, many skin conditions require other medical or surgical treatment.

▶ If you have been treated with the anti-acne drug Accutane (oral Isotretinoin), you may heal more slowly than the average patient and be at increased risk for scarring. Accutane suppresses acne by shutting down oil production in the sebaceous glands, making the skin dry, extremely fragile and impairing its ability to regenerate new epidermal cells. Because of this, some doctors recommend waiting at least a year after Accutane therapy has ended before considering laser resurfacing.

▶ Inform your doctor if you have ever had a cold sore, a herpes infection or shingles. Laser resurfacing can reactivate the viruses that cause these conditions, making them flare up again.

Most of the measures doctors take to prepare skin for laser resurfacing surgery are done in anticipation of problems that could crop up afterwards, during the healing period.

Because raw, newly lased skin is extremely vulnerable to microbes, some doctors prescribe an antibiotic at the time of surgery to provide resistance against possible bacterial infections. Lased skin is also highly susceptible to the herpes simplex virus, even in patients who have never had a herpes infection or cold sore. Herpes can delay healing and lead to scarring. To prevent this, most doctors now routinely prescribe an oral antiviral medication such as acyclovir to all patients undergoing full-face resurfacing, starting at the time of surgery and continuing for seven to 10 days afterwards.

A very common postoperative complication is temporary skin darkening (transient hyperpigmentation) in which the lased areas turn noticeably more brown than the surrounding skin. Although most frequently seen in people with naturally dark complexions, transient hyperpigmentation can also occur in very fair-skinned individuals. Because of this some doctors like to pretreat their patients with skin lightening creams starting several weeks before surgery.

In addition to these preoperative preparations, some physicians are experimentally pre-treating skin with topical vitamin solutions that may help speed healing and cut down on the period of prolonged redness that typically follows laser surgery. Some studies suggest that increasing the skin's natural store of certain vitamins may boost its ability to heal.

Laser resurfacing is an outpatient procedure, usually performed at the physician's office. It does not require general anesthesia. But if a large area such as the entire face is to be lased, the doctor may want to use a strong intravenous sedative, and you will be asked not to eat or drink for six hours before the scheduled surgery. When you go in, wear comfortable clothes—nothing that you have to pull over your head to remove or put back on—and come with a friend or relative who can drive you home.

At the doctor's office, your face will be scrubbed bare of all traces of makeup and soil. You will probably be given a local anesthetic and perhaps a mild sedative as well. A topical analgesic cream may be rubbed over the skin to numb it before the local anesthetic is injected in the areas that will be treated.

Because the laser beam represents a potentially serious hazard to the eyes, everyone in the laser room is required to wear special protective glasses. Your eyes will be covered with opaque plastic goggles or thick, moistened gauze pads. If the skin around the eyes is to be treated, metal shields, like contact lenses, will be placed directly on the eyes with their edges beneath the lids.

HOW SKIN IS LASED

The laser beam, measured out in intense precise pulses, is delivered through a hand-held device attached to the end of an articulated arm like that on a dentist's drill. The beam cannot be seen, but its effects are instantly visible. It hits the skin with a faint, but distinctly audible sound—a high, thin combination of pop and fizz. Instantly, a tiny puff of steam containing vaporized skin cells appears. Called the laser plume, this substance is sucked away by a special vacuuming device. Some partially vaporized cells remain on the skin as a fine white ashy substance.

Controlled by a mechanism built into the hand piece, the light strikes as a rapid-fire series of pulses laid down in a small geometric pattern no larger than the tip of a finger. Each succession of pulses leaves a white circle or square comprised of desiccated skin cells. In short order, a section of skin several inches square is covered with little patterns of skin detritus. (The hand piece may also be adjusted to produce other patterns, or even single pulses, to cover differently contoured areas of the face.) The surgeon then wipes them away with damp gauze, uncovering a shiny, pink smoothness. Then the beam is moved over other parts of the face, until the skin is stripped of its surface.

Deep wrinkles require several passes of the laser beam. So after an entire skin section has been lased, the doctor generally goes over it once or twice again—several more times in areas like the cheeks where the skin is relatively thick—as if peeling an onion one layer at a time.

If you are not having a full-face resurfacing procedure, the doctor will work in what are known as cosmetic units—broad areas, such as the entire cheek or forehead, that encompass and extend well beyond the targeted wrinkles. The laser peel should get progressively shallower toward the edges of the cosmetic unit, so that the treated skin blends into the surrounding areas. A physician who merely traces a wrinkle with the laser beam will leave an obvious depression and a line of demarcation.

Patients who are having their entire faces lased usually don't feel a thing because, as a rule, they are so heavily sedated. However, those who are only having small areas treated sometimes find the procedure quite painful. Because of the difficulty in reaching some facial nerves with a local anesthetic, all the areas that are to be lased cannot always be totally numbed, and those sections may hurt as the work is done.

After surgery, the lased areas will almost immediately start to swell and become extremely sensitive. You will probably be sent home with your face thickly coated with a healing ointment, in an attempt to shield the injured surface and to guard against infection. Some doctors like to cover the face with semi-occlusive dressings—thin, gel-like bandages that cling to and soothe the raw surface.

If you have had a full-face resurfacing procedure you will feel terrible and look just as bad. You probably won't want anyone to see you for four or five days. The swelling peaks in 24 to 48 hours, and your face may look truly grotesque—a flattened-out moon shape, hugely swollen and bright red. Your eyes will be reduced to slits and it will hurt to open your mouth, making it difficult to speak or eat.

Smaller areas will be almost as swollen and painful as larger ones. "I looked like Daffy Duck," grimaced one patient, who had laser surgery around her mouth. "A goon from outer space" is how another woman described her appearance after resurfacing around the mouth and eyes.

Within 24 hours, the skin will start to ooze a thin, clear, yellowish serum. Left to itself, this liquid hardens into a thick, rigid crust, much like a big scab. This is a natural, self-protective reaction on the part of your injured skin. But a thick crust not only feels extremely uncomfortable, it can also interfere with healing or cause the skin to heal unevenly. Liberal use of wet compresses will dissolve the hardened serum and keep a heavy crust from forming. Do not try to pick off any areas where hard crusts develop; this could lead to a scar.

The swelling usually starts to go down in two or three days—although your skin will still be raw and painfully sensitive to the touch. By the fourth or fifth day the oozing should stop. Your doctor will want to see you by the third or fourth day to check your progress. If you have any areas of hard, stubborn crusting, a nurse or aide may gently soak or steam them off.

During this period, and for a week or more beyond, you will look as if you have a very bad sunburn—or worse. "I looked like I had been in some horrible accident, like an explosion or something," remembered Rosemary, 68, of the aftermath of laser resurfacing around her mouth and between her eyes. "I went shopping with my husband six days afterward, and people looked truly shocked. I just know they were saying, 'That poor lady. She must have been severely burned.'"

Do not try to treat the red areas of your skin with anything other than the medications or ointments your doctor has recommended or prescribed. The laser has exposed the live cells deep in the dermis, leaving them extremely vulnerable to the many possible allergens that all over-the-counter topical analgesics, burn lotions, moisturizers and cleansing agents contain. You can get a severe allergic reaction to any one of these ingredients, even if you have never been allergic to a cosmetic product in the past. Even "natural" products such as aloe and vitamin E oil have produced irritation or allergic reactions in laser-treated skin.

Any oral antibiotics or antiviral medicines your doctor has prescribed will continue through the first week. For large skin surface areas, some surgeons also advise the use of oral corticosteroids to help reduce swelling and inflammation. Medications to alleviate pain and help you sleep are also usually needed during the early healing stage (the first week).

It takes an average of seven to 10 days for the skin to re-epithelialize, that is, to build up a new layer of surface cells. After that, your face may feel drier than usual for several weeks.

This is because the treated skin is still healing and unable to retain moisture as it normally does. You may experience mild peeling; your skin may appear chapped and flaky. It also may itch. And you may break out in small acne-like bumps and pimples, especially if you have acne-prone skin. If any of these things happen, inform your doctor, who will prescribe medication to control the problem. Again, do not try to treat it yourself.

If you are accustomed to regular exercise, wait a week or 10 days and then resume your workouts slowly. Stick to light activities at first. Anything that might cause you to perspire heavily or to grunt or grimace can burst the fragile new blood vessels in your face. Wait three to four weeks before resuming strenuous exercise such as aerobics, weight training or competitive sports. And don't smoke. Nicotine constricts the blood vessels in your face, depriving your skin of the oxygen it needs for optimum healing.

You will have to wear a strong sunscreen with an SPF of 20 or more every day during this period and for the following three months or so. While your skin is still healing, it is abnormally vulnerable to solar radiation and you will be prone to serious burning. And even minimal exposure to ultraviolet light can cause permanent alterations in your skin color.

Your skin color may change in any case. It is very common for the lased areas to darken and turn brown, starting three to four weeks after the surgery; this happens to as many as one-third of all patients treated with the CO_2 laser. Again, if you notice it happening to you, tell your doctor right away. A topical cream containing a skin-lightening chemical such as hydroquinone can arrest the pigment changes, and will usually lighten the brown marks within three or four weeks. Without treatment, it can take up to a year for the skin to gradually return to its original tone.

SERIOUS THINGS TO LOOK OUT FOR

You will have to take a few extra precautions if your doctor has put bandages on your face. The semi-occlusive dressings that some doctors like to use will protect the raw skin, soak up extruded serum and help maintain a moist environment that aids in healing. But dressings can also cause some problems. The most important thing to remember is that you cannot pull them off. Most are designed to stay on until the skin re-epithelializes.

Your doctor will probably want to see you the day after the operation to change the dressings. After that, they should stay in place until the skin has replaced the missing surface cells—a process that may take another seven to 10 days. Because bandages can start to get uncomfortable or annoying during this period, some patients get tempted to pick them off. But doing so can disrupt the new epithelial cells, which will delay healing and may even lead to a scar. Unless the bandages fall off on their own, leave them on until your next doctor's visit. They will be removed after your skin has been checked.

Sometimes, dressings—by covering and blocking pores—will cause acne-like breakouts. In other cases, they may contribute to the formation of adhesions—tiny areas where the swollen skin is held in small folds and two surfaces adhere. Neither of these are serious problems if they are attended to promptly. If you break out, your doctor will start you on an anti-acne regimen. Skin adhesions can be quickly and painlessly released in the office, and the skin will proceed to heal normally.

Whether your skin has been bandaged or not, it will be abnormally susceptible to infection for several weeks after the operation. Candida (yeast), herpes and staph infections are particular dangers; all can cause skin changes that may result in a scar. Call your doctor instantly if you develop any signs of infection such as a high fever, severe localized pain, swelling (after the initial swelling has subsided), or any kind of blistering or discharge other than the clear oozing typical of the first few days.

The most serious potential complication of laser resurfacing is the development of a raised (hypertrophic) scar. The first signs of hypertrophic scarring commonly appear three to four weeks after the operation, often in areas where there is much natural movement, such as around the mouth. The first hint is usually intense redness; the skin in one area becomes a much deeper color than its surroundings. If you gently touch the red section with your fingertips, you may feel an underlying hardness or stiffness. If the skin around the mouth is involved, you may not be able to open it fully.

Let your doctor know right away if you notice either redness or hardening in any part of your lased skin. If caught early enough, a hypertrophic scar can often be prevented from getting larger and, with treatment, could flatten. If the scar is allowed to fully form, it is likely to be permanent—although there are other laser techniques that can improve its appearance (see Chapter 9).

THE LONG TERM OUTLOOK

Your treated skin should appear substantially healed in four to six weeks. However, it will still be changing. The redness will turn to pink, which will persist for a few more months. Although you won't be able to tell from looking at your face or touching it, there may be a small amount of residual swelling. This can temporarily give your skin an abnormally smooth, glassy appearance.

You can also expect your skin to look and feel excessively tight for at least six weeks and probably longer, due to shrinkage of the collagen fibers in the dermis. Some people find this uncomfortable, particularly around the eyes where the skin is thin and delicate. In some cases—especially if a patient has had a previous eye lift—the skin around the eyes may tighten so much that part of the inner lids turn out. This condition, called ectropion, may subside over the following three to five months as the skin gradually relaxes.

Over the same period, some wrinkles will reappear. Commonly, it is the dynamic wrinkles—especially those from the nose to the corners of the mouth, between the eyes and across the forehead—that come back, although they tend to be far less obvious than they were before surgery.

On close inspection your skin will probably look more pink than usual for some time—anywhere from six months to a year after surgery. This is because new blood vessels are growing and developing. In some people, perceptible pinkness lasts well beyond a year, although it may only be noticeable during heavy exertion.

Because this lingering color sometimes annoys patients, some doctors offer to treat the superficial blood vessels with the same laser used on other skin-reddening conditions such as rosacea (see Chapter 8). However, it is far better to simply leave the skin alone, allowing it to heal normally at its own snail's pace. In the long run your skin will be smoother and firmer because the new blood vessels are playing an important role in rebuilding the dermis and its collagen support network.

All told, your skin's ultimate post-surgical condition—what surgeons call the "steady-state"—will probably not be apparent until the full year has passed.

SKIN CARE FOLLOWING LASER RESURFACING

During the first two weeks after surgery—when your skin first oozes, crusts and swells for several days and then becomes abnormally tender and very vulnerable to injury—you must try to control the pain and swelling and allow the skin to heal with as little interference as possible. Here are some basic techniques:

1. To reduce swelling and alleviate pain, keep cloth-wrapped ice packs or commercially available flexible cold gel packs on the laser-treated areas for three days after surgery. (Packages of frozen peas or corn make excellent substitutes; they are cheap, readily available, and conform easily to the shape of the face.) Apply the ice packs for at least 10 to 15 minutes at a time every hour while awake.

2. Keep your head elevated and as immobile as possible when sleeping or resting. Sleep propped up on pillows. Some people find it helpful to sleep in a recliner for the first few nights.

3. Take acetaminophen (such as Tylenol) if necessary to bolster the effects of any prescribed pain medication. Aspirin is not recommended because it can enhance bleeding tendencies.

4. Frequently, at least once every one to two hours, gently apply wet compresses to your skin to dissolve and soak off oozing serum. Use a soft washcloth or gauze dipped in cool water. (Use a fresh cloth each time; re-applying the same ones could lead to an infection.) Do not pick off hardened crusts; if they are not removed with soaking, leave them alone.

5. Between soakings and applications of ice packs, keep the skin well coated with whatever protective ointment your doctor has prescribed. Keeping the skin moist in this fashion speeds healing because new skin cells tend to grow faster in a moist environment.

6. On the fourth day, you may attempt to wash your skin twice a day with a mild soap-free cleanser (e.g. Catrix Correction Cream Wash, Cetaphil or Aquanil). If you feel a burning sensation when you wash, wait another day or two before using the cleanser again.

7. By the end of the first week, you will have seen your doctor for at least one follow-up visit and probably been told when you can start using moisturizer, sunscreen and foundation makeup—usually sometime between the first and second week. Your doctor will either supply or recommend products which don't contain additives that provoke acne or allergies. Your sunscreen should have a Sun Protection Factor (SPF) of at least 15. Most physicians encourage the use of a SPF of 25 to 30.

To avoid an allergic reaction to cosmetic ingredients, wait until your skin has re-epithelialized (usually by the tenth day postoperatively) to apply makeup. By then, your face will have a new layer of protective surface cells, although it will still be extremely sensitive and very red.

Laser surgery clinics often supply patients with special camouflage makeup to wear for the first four to six weeks following resurfacing. (Two common brands are Covermark and Dermablend, available at some large department stores, as well as through physicians.) These masking cosmetics, originally designed to conceal disfiguring scars or birthmarks, are thick, oil-based formulations containing greater-than-average amounts of pigment. Those used to cover red discolorations are often tinted green to counteract the redness. They take some skill to apply. Usually they are patted on over the red areas, set with a special powder and then covered with regular foundation.

Unfortunately, camouflage cosmetics are very occlusive and can cause acne in some individuals. Even when expertly applied, they can look somewhat mask-like. And many patients dislike the way they feel. For these reasons, some people prefer conventional foundation. Most major cosmetic companies have heavy versions of their ordinary foundation cosmetics. One product that has proven popular with a number of laser patients is Estee Lauder's Maximum Coverage Lightweight Makeup. Acne-prone individuals have liked Clinique's Continuous Coverage foundation. Both are available at department stores. These cosmetics won't hide the red, but they will tone it down to an acceptable level. Most people will just think you spent a little too much time at the beach.

Whatever makeup you use, be sure to first protect your skin with the moisturizer or sunscreen your doctor has recommended. And be particularly gentle when you remove your makeup; rubbing hard will retard healing and can lead to permanent changes in your skin's texture.

The most common complication following laser surgery is temporary skin darkening—called **transient post-inflammatory hyperpigmentation**—in which the lased areas turn noticeably more brown or tan than the surrounding skin. The condition is not permanent, but it can persist for many months or even years if the skin is exposed to sunlight. Any patient may experience post-inflammatory hyperpigmentation to some degree, but it is most frequently seen on people with olive or darker complexions.

People owe their skin color to the brown pigment **melanin**, a chemical compound created in the lowest (basal) layer of the epidermis by special cells called **melanocytes**. Melanocytes synthesize melanin inside microscopic packages called **melanosomes** and then transfer them to other skin cells, the **keratinocytes**. Everyone, no matter what skin color, has about the same number of melanocytes—in a ratio of roughly one melanocyte to every six keratinocytes. It is the size of the melanosomes and the way they are distributed that account for racial differences in skin color. In general, melanosomes are larger in dark skin and smaller in light skin.

Melanin, in addition to determining skin color, is the body's first line of defense against destructive sunlight, functioning as a filter against ultraviolet rays. This complex chemical may also act in some way to ward off certain toxins and to counteract the damaging effects of free oxygen radicals. Any assault on the skin—particularly any injury that causes the skin to become inflamed—can trigger the melanocytes to step up their production of protective melanin. This is what causes a suntan, the most familiar form of post-inflammatory hyperpigmentation.

The manner in which skin produces melanin in response to

sunlight determines the classifications into which dermatologists group skin. There are six of these so-called **photo-types**:

Type I: Very fair, milky, often freckled skin, with blond or red hair and blue or green eyes. Always burns, never tans. Usually becomes increasingly more freckled in response to the sun—evidently because the skin is so inefficient in producing melanin and can only do so in tiny patches.

Type II: Pale, lightly pigmented skin, with blond to brown hair and blue, green or brown eyes. Burns first, then tans with some freckling.

Type III: Medium-toned olive or beige skin. Brown to black hair and usually brown eyes. Occasionally burns, tans well and rarely freckles.

Type IV: Dark olive to light brown skin, brown to black hair, brown eyes. Rarely burns, tans quickly and darkly. Never freckles.

Type V: Medium to dark brown skin, dark brown to black hair, brown eyes. Never burns, always tans.

Type VI: Very dark brown to black skin, black hair and dark brown or black eyes. Never burns, always tans, although the tan is imperceptible because the base skin tone is so dark.

Physicians still do not fully understand how or why it occurs, but the melanocytes in dark skin tend to respond more rapidly and efficiently to ultraviolet light and to injury. Although there are exceptions, it is axiomatic that people with skin types I and II (the poor tanners) rarely experience post-inflammatory hyperpigmentation. Types III and above usually do. This is why many laser surgeons are reluctant to resurface patients with naturally dark skin. However, as doctors have become more familiar with lasers and with the ins and outs of postoperative care, more experienced laser surgeons have started to treat darker skin types.

The first step is careful preoperative evaluation. People who have shown hyperpigmentation in the past in response to an injury (even a healing pimple or insect bite) are likely to have a similar response to the laser. Many doctors put these patients on a preoperative regimen of topical skin lightening medication containing **hydroquinone**, a chemical that acts on melanocytes to inhibit melanin synthesis. Theoretically, lessening the all-over melanin content in an area will help minimize the effect of subsequent pigment overproduction in that spot.

More importantly, people who are considered at particular risk for hyperpigmentation are cautioned to be fanatically careful about avoiding the sun after surgery. They are advised to stay inside as much as possible, wear hats and other sun-protective clothing, and to make liberal use of broad-spectrum sunscreen containing agents that block both UVA and UVB radiation—even indoors. Sunlight through a window pane can trigger hyperpigmentation in susceptible individuals. Some reports suggest that even light from fluorescent bulbs may do it.

If hyperpigmentation is going to occur, it usually appears within three to four weeks after surgery—although it can develop several months afterward. As soon as the skin starts to darken, the patient is prescribed a skin lightening cream which contains a strong concentration of hydroquinone, in some cases supplemented with other bleaching substances. If this topical therapy is started at the first sign of browning, and the patient is consistent in using the cream, the dark areas should lighten within four weeks or so. Application of a mild acid (a superficial chemical peel) four weeks after surgery and repeated one to two weeks later, may help speed the lightening process by removing melanin-containing skin cells in the upper epidermis.

Left to itself, hyperpigmentation following laser surgery usually clears up in about a year—if the skin is completely protected from the sun. But if the lased areas are exposed to any significant amount of sunlight during that period, ultraviolet radiation may actually alter the pigmentary mechanism, and the hyperpigmentation can become permanent.

A related reason for caution in using the laser on darkly pigmented skin is the fear of **hypopigmentation** or skin lightening. In areas where the skin is injured very deeply, normal melanocytes sometimes do not regenerate. No melanin is subsequently produced and the skin in that spot appears white.

Permanent hypopigmentation is a common side effect of deep chemical peels, and to a somewhat lesser extent, of dermabrasion. It is a very rare and totally unpredictable complication in laser resurfacing surgery. It occurs in less than one percent of patients and appears to be unrelated to skin type. Type VI skin is apparently at no more at risk than Type I. But, because a white patch is far more noticeable on dark skin, the consequences are more serious for people with naturally dark skin.

Hypopigmentation shows up on a delayed basis, several months to a year after surgery. A prudent step to rule out the chance of hypopigmentation on very dark skin is to lase a small test spot in an inconspicuous location, and wait six to 12 months to gauge the long-term response.

C H A P T E R T H R E E

SMOOTHING OUT ACNE SCARS

"*W*hen I look back on it, I realize that the defining issue of my life was my skin," said Emily, who at 41, underwent laser resurfacing surgery for severe acne scars that had marred her features her entire adult life. "The kinds of things you're dealing with when you have acne are very different from what people go through when they have crow's feet or wrinkles or whatever. Acne is a huge self-esteem issue. Because you know, when you don't even want to look at your own face, that's pretty significant."

Emily's feeling are echoed by thousands of other patients who suffer from serious acne and the often disfiguring facial scars that can result from it. Many say that self-consciousness about their appearance has dominated their lives, undermining their self-esteem and casting a cloud over personal and professional relationships. As 26-year-old Alison, who endured an acne-plagued adolescence and young adulthood put it, "The scars go far deeper than the skin."

TINA ALSTER, M.D. & LYDIA PRESTON

In fact, acne scars go deeply into the physical structure of the skin as well. This is what makes them so obvious in appearance, and it is why they are so difficult to eradicate.

Acne begins inside the hair follicles, in the skin's middle layer, the dermis. Tiny sebaceous glands lie to the side of each follicle, producing oil (sebum). In normal skin, sebum travels freely up the hair shaft along with other cellular fluids, "washing out" natural debris such as dead cells, and bathing the surface of the skin in a thin, protective, natural moisturizer.

For a complex set of reasons that doctors still do not fully understand, this mechanism malfunctions in acne-prone individuals and some follicles become blocked with a plug of cellular debris. A plug high up in the follicle with its top exposed is called an open comedone, or blackhead. A plug beneath the surface of the skin is a closed comedone, or whitehead.

A pimple forms when trapped oil and additional debris in the follicle are attacked by bacteria. This causes what is, in effect, a small infection. Eventually the blocked follicle bursts from built-up pressure, spilling its contents into surrounding tissue and spreading the infectious material deep into the dermis. The result is an inflamed pustule or cyst that acts to destroy a portion of the dermis and its network of collagen fibers.

When one of these destructive lesions heals, it can leave one of two kinds of scars behind. The skin may react to the damage by overproducing collagen. The result is a raised, or hypertrophic, scar. More commonly, the collagen in the area grows back only partially or not at all, leaving a depressed, or atrophic, scar. (Chickenpox and certain injuries or surgical procedures can also leave atrophic scars.) Atrophic acne scars range in size and shape from wide, saucer-like craters to narrow, deep pits that make the skin look as if it has been jabbed with an ice pick.

Over the years, doctors have tried to smooth out atrophic acne scars with many of the same surgical techniques used on wrinkles, including dermabrasion, chemical peels, and injections of filler materials such as silicone, collagen or fat. In a technique called punch grafting, a little core of skin containing a single scar is cut out with a metal hole punch, and a tiny plug of skin—usually taken from behind the ear—is put in to fill out the cavity. Unfortunately none of these methods commonly used to eradicate acne scars has ever been regarded as fully successful—as most acne-scarred patients in search of a smoother complexion discover.

"I looked into just about everything, and tried most of them," said Emily. "Absolutely nothing worked. My skin was too bad for a chemical peel. Every doctor I ever talked to said it wouldn't do any good. Collagen was OK, I guess, but it wears off. And then I started reading things that made me concerned about side effects, so I stopped doing it." Emily also tried punch grafting ("that just gave me another kind of scar") and dermabrasion. "That was the worst. It was horrible to go through and I felt it made my scars look worse."

Injections with filler agents such as collagen or fat are effective for only a limited period of time; eventually the body absorbs the injected material and the depression returns. Sometimes injections make the scars look even more obvious. This is because the walls of depressed scars are typically lined in tough fibrous tissue, making them stiffer in texture than the surrounding skin. Filler agents sometimes push up the surrounding skin, creating a kind of doughnut effect around the core.

Moreover, because acne pits form deep in the dermis, atrophic acne scars commonly extend below the level where skin can be removed safely by resurfacing techniques such as dermabrasion or chemical peels. As with deep wrinkles, only very deep chemical peels or extremely aggressive dermabrasion has any appreciable effect. Scarring and pigment changes are common complications.

Elaine, who at the age of 25 had dermabrasion for acne scars, wound up with dead white, porcelain cheeks. Although she was pleased by the improvement in the texture of her skin— her deep scars had become shallow depressions—the unnaturally pale color was disturbing. "I mean those cheeks are WHITE," she said 15 years later.

The prospect of winding up with results like Elaine's and Emily's frightened many acne patients away from scar treatment. Concluding that none of the available therapies were worth the risk, 36-year-old Patricia resigned herself to living with her scars. "I knew there was nothing I could do and they were never going to go away. So I made my peace with it."

Dennis—who after investigating and rejecting all of the available scar revision treatments, grew a beard to hide his scarred cheeks—was slightly more optimistic. "I've always figured that some day medical science would come up with something better," he said.

LASER RESURFACING FOR ACNE SCARS

For many people, laser resurfacing with the new high energy pulsed carbon dioxide laser has proved to be that something better—a safer, generally more effective alternative to conventional remedies for atrophic acne scars. (Hypertrophic scars are treated with a different laser technique; see Chapter 9.)

It is not usually the means to a flawless complexion. Most acne scars cannot be completely eradicated by any technique. The chief advantage of laser treatment over other resurfacing methods is that the laser's precision allows the most improvement possible with the least risk. An experienced laser surgeon can peel as deeply as feasible into the dermis in order to have the maximum possible impact without compromising the skin's ability to regenerate a normal new surface.

Controlled studies have shown that laser resurfacing may effect a 50 to 100 percent improvement in the appearance of atrophic acne scars (the latter figure meaning that they totally disappear). Success depends greatly on how deep and fibrous the scars are to begin with. Shallow, soft saucer-like depressions respond the best; tough, fibrous ice-pick scars are the most resistant to treatment. Patients with extremely deep or extensive scarring often undergo two resurfacing operations, usually spaced at least nine to 12 months apart in order for the skin to fully heal after the first procedure. Typically they see the most dramatic changes following the first treatment, and more subtle, yet still measurable improvements after the second.

The procedure is identical to that described in the preceding chapter for wrinkles (pages 36-37). All of the same precautions and preoperative routines listed on pages 32-36 also apply, with a few additional considerations specific to acne patients.

▶ If you have active acne, your doctor will want to get it under control first with Retin-A, glycolic acid or antibiotics. Lasing inflamed acne pimples may increase the chances of complications such as long-term pigment changes or scars.

▶ Remember, doctors do not recommend undergoing laser resurfacing within a year, or more, of treatment with the oral anti-acne drug isotretinoin (Accutane) which suppresses sebaceous gland activity, making skin dry, extremely fragile and more prone to scarring.

▶ As with wrinkles, past treatment with injectable collagen, silicone or other filler agents may have caused underlying fibrosis which can alter the effect of the laser light. And skin that has been subjected to deep dermabrasion or a chemical peel is more than normally prone to lasting pigment changes following laser surgery.

▶ Because of the increased risk of scarring in those areas of the body, the resurfacing laser cannot be used on the back or on the neck, where many people have additional acne scars. Doctors can treat those areas with light to medium depth chemical peels that will improve the texture of the skin somewhat while making the skin closer in color to the more aggressively lased areas on the face.

▶ A possible concern for older patients: In the past, serious acne was sometimes treated with x-rays—a strategy now supplanted by safer, more effective therapies. If you had radiation treatment for acne when you were younger, be sure to discuss it with your doctor. X-rays make permanent changes in skin cells which could affect the way your skin heals, and put you at increased risk for scarring.

WHAT YOU CAN EXPECT

The healing period following laser resurfacing for acne is the same as that described on pages 38–41, starting with intense swelling, oozing and crusting and progressing to the deep red sunburned look that lasts for many weeks afterward.

Long-term results vary widely, depending on a number of factors, from the skill of the surgeon to individual differences among patients. "I guess I have to say it wasn't as successful as

I hoped it would be," confessed Dennis a month after undergoing the procedure. "I can see some improvement. But it was a lot to go through. And I think I'm still going to want to grow my beard back."

Other patients find that the shallower, less obvious indentations that remain following resurfacing make a significant improvement in their appearance. "It was a real ordeal, but it was worth it," said Alison. "I used to look in a mirror and all I could see were the pock marks. Now I look and I can see that they're still there, but it's hard to find them. They're not the first thing you notice." Like a good many patients, Alison also noted a change in the overall texture and quality of her complexion. "My skin really felt rejuvenated. Before, it always seemed a little rough and irritated; now it's softer and more supple."

As with resurfacing for wrinkles, a large part of whatever changes occur seems to be due to alterations in the collagen fibers of the dermis. The general tightening and remodeling of collagen that occurs after laser resurfacing fills in and smooths out the skin over a period of months. Some people notice that their skin continues to gradually change and improve for as much as a year or longer following surgery.

For many women, the mark of success is freedom from the heavy makeup that many of them have worn for years to cover up their scars. Noted Emily, who underwent two laser resurfacing operations, "I almost never wear face makeup anymore. When I do, it's because I want a more finished look; it's not a camouflage thing."

"I feel my skin is dramatically better," said Katherine, 42, who relied for years on heavy pancake makeup to cover the scars left by a short but severe bout of acne at the age of 35. "Makeup used to dominate my life. Every few hours, I would just drop everything and go fix my face. Now I don't even think about it."

"There's just no comparison," concluded Emily. "My husband always claimed that my skin never bothered him. But now he keeps commenting on just how beautiful it looks. Honestly, I have nice skin. I mean I don't have perfect skin. Who does? But the improvement is amazing."

SKIN CARE AFTER LASER RESURFACING FOR ACNE SCARS

1. To reduce swelling and alleviate pain during the first three or four days after surgery, while the swollen, lased areas are oozing and crusting, put cloth-wrapped ice packs or cold gel packs on the treated skin. (Packages of frozen peas or corn which easily conform to the face are a handy and economical substitute.) Apply the ice packs for at least 10 to 15 minutes at a time every hour while awake.

2. To further reduce swelling, keep your head elevated when sleeping or resting.

3. Take the pain medications prescribed by your doctor. If necessary, take acetaminophen (Tylenol) to bolster the pain relief.

4. Every one to two hours, gently apply wet compresses to your skin to dissolve and soak off oozing serum. Use a soft washcloth or gauze dipped in cool water. (Use a fresh cloth each time; re-applying the same ones could lead to an infection.)

5. Between soakings and icings, keep the skin well coated with the protective ointment your doctor has prescribed. Do not use any over-the-counter analgesic preparation or moisturizer; they may cause serious allergic reactions in your raw skin. And be on the alert for small white bumps (milia) or other breakouts; the occlusive ointments and dressings which help speed healing by keeping the skin moist can also cause acne-prone skin to break out. If this happens to you, notify your doctor.

6. On the fourth day, start washing your skin twice a day with a mild soap-free cleanser (e.g. Catrix Correction Cream Wash, Cetaphil or Aquanil). If you feel a burning sensation when you wash, wait another day or two before using the cleanser again to allow more time for your skin to heal.

7. After getting the go-ahead from your doctor, start using moisturizer, sunscreen and foundation makeup—usually sometime between the first and second week. The doctor will either supply or recommend products without additives that could cause allergic reactions or acne breakouts.

8. Use a non-occlusive makeup (e.g. Clinique Continuous Coverage) over your moisturizer or sunscreen. Be very careful when removing your makeup; rubbing hard will retard healing and can lead to permanent changes in your skin's texture or effect a scar.

CHAPTER FOUR

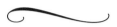

THINGS THAT GO BUMP:
WARTS, TAGS, MOLES AND OTHER SKIN GROWTHS

*E*dward was a keen outdoorsman and it was written all over his face. By the time he was 50, his weathered, leathery skin appeared permanently ruddy. His cheeks, nose and forehead were rough with scaly, irregularly shaped reddish bumps. And his lips had the sunburned, chapped look common to skiers, sailors, climbers and others who have spent years working or playing in the glare of the sun and its reflection off oceans or snow-covered mountains.

Arnold's skin told a different story —in his case, a far from accurate one. Arnold, 62, had never been more than a moderate social drinker. But his florid face and large, bulbous red nose made him look like the popular conception of a falling-down drunk. As he himself ruefully noted, his nose bore a striking resemblance to that of stereotypical screen inebriate W.C. Fields.

Rebecca had another set of skin problems. During two pregnancies, she reported, her skin had seemed to go berserk, breaking out with dozens of bright red, pinpoint-sized bumps and a host of little flesh-colored projections called skin tags. As she approached her mid-40s, she began to see something else— small horny growths that looked as if they had been stuck on from the outside. "It seems like the older I get, the more THINGS I get on me," she exclaimed in exasperation.

Most people do. Very few of us are blessed with absolutely flawless skin. And even those who are eventually acquire a few "things" over the years — little bumps or growths, small scaly patches or strange discolorations. Very often, they are manifestations of advancing age, "senile degradation" of the skin, as it is sometimes called. This simply means that as people get older, their skin cells do not always function as well as they did in youth; as they reproduce, aging cells tend to periodically produce odd little anomalies. Sun damage and hormonal changes, such as those that occur in pregnancy or menopause, can have a similar effect. And sometimes, things just appear on the skin for no apparent reason at all.

Together, Edward, Arnold and Rebecca presented a representative sample of the some of the more common ones. People typically refer to them as "moles" or "warts." That's often what they look like, and sometimes, that's exactly what they are. In other cases, they are any one of a host of other surface disorders that fall into the very large general category of superficial skin growths or tumors.

Although patients become concerned, even panicky, when they hear the words "growth" or "tumor," the terms do not necessarily imply that a condition is serious. Most common skin tumors are completely harmless, although some have the potential for developing into skin cancers and others may be the sign of an underlying disease that requires treatment. And some, even if they are not harmful in themselves, can cause local irritation or pain if they are in a place where they press on surrounding tissues or get rubbed by a piece of clothing.

But for the most part, skin growths are objectionable simply because they are unsightly and indicative of age. For most people, that is more than enough reason to want them taken off.

TARGETING SKIN GROWTHS WITH LASERS

Removing superficial skin tumors was one of the first ways lasers were employed in medicine. As early as the 1960s, dermatologists were using carbon dioxide lasers to vaporize many kinds of growths. But doctors soon became disenchanted with laser skin surgery because it was so difficult to control the thermal impact of the first generation, continuous wave lasers. Heat from the laser beam built up quickly in the skin, spreading beyond the targeted lesions and frequently burning healthy skin to the point of actually charring it.

Today's more precise, tissue-specific pulsed lasers offer an expanding range of safe and effective ways to remove skin tumors. Many doctors now regard laser resurfacing as the treatment of choice for badly sun-damaged skin like Edward's, roughened by solar lesions known as actinic keratoses and by a condition called actinic chelitis in which the lips become chronically inflamed and scaly from overexposure to the sun. Laser surgery has also been proven to be the most effective means of re-contouring the nodular swelling on noses like Arthur's, distorted by a condition called rhinophyma, which is often seen in advanced stages of rosacea. Other typical candidates for laser removal include moles, skin tags, warts and scaly seborrheic keratoses (Rebecca's horny little bumps).

Laser surgeons have several options when it comes to removing these and a number of other, less common growths.

Many benign, superficial skin tumors can easily be removed with a pulsed carbon dioxide laser, the same high powered laser used to resurface wrinkled or acne-scarred skin. The laser vaporizes the abnormal cells that comprise the tumors, leaving adjacent skin unaffected.

Other lasers, those that target structures beneath the skin, work by destroying some critical constituent of a growth. What are broadly classified as pigment-specific lasers destroy cells containing the skin pigment melanin. They are used on brown spots, such as freckles, sun spots, brown birthmarks and most moles (Chapter 5), and are also used to remove tattoos (Chapter 6). Vascular-specific lasers, such as those discussed in Chapters 7 and 8, destroy blood vessels. These are used on red growths, from disfiguring red birthmarks to minor "cherry spots" —the little red bumps that popped up on Rebecca during pregnancy.

Whichever laser treatment is being contemplated, any skin growth targeted for removal should first be evaluated by a dermatologist. There are a bewildering variety of small skin tumors and many of them resemble one another so closely that they can only be told apart by laboratory examination. A number of pre-cancerous lesions, and even some skin cancers, look very much like harmless growths—and vice versa. Because only a few superficial cancers and pre-cancers can be removed safely with a laser, any suspicion of malignancy calls for a pre-surgical biopsy.

The growths described in this chapter are the most common of those that are now frequently treated with the pulsed CO_2 laser. They are all essentially superficial tumors that are either confined entirely to the epidermis or that reach only partially into the dermis, just below. The time-honored techniques for removing these tumors include shaving or excision with a scalpel, dermabrasion, freezing with liquid nitrogen, or burning with an electric needle or various acids. Except when employed on the smallest and most superficial growths, all of these conventional methods for removing skin tumors tend to produce scars or to permanently alter the skin's color or texture.

The pulsed CO_2 laser is far less likely to leave any kind of permanent mark. The procedure is, in effect, a kind of highly selective resurfacing operation, similar to that described in detail in Chapter 2. The laser beam vaporizes the abnormal tissue and the skin rebuilds the area with normal skin cells, creating a smooth, unblemished surface. Done correctly, the procedure leaves little or no scarring to mark the spot where the unsightly growth once was.

Because the laser beam instantly seals blood vessels and little lymph structures, it works bloodlessly and does not initially cause swelling. Surgeons can see clearly as they operate, allowing them to be very precise in determining how much tissue to remove. Patients tend to heal quickly and with little discomfort. Moreover, laser surgery is usually faster than other methods, a boon when operating on patients with multiple lesions. (It is not unusual for people to have 100 or more little growths that they want to have taken off all at once.) And the laser is extremely thorough—less likely to leave parts of a lesion behind to "seed" new growth and cause the tumor to eventually reappear.

BENIGN EPIDERMAL GROWTHS

Those benign superficial growths that are confined entirely to the surface layer of the skin (the epidermis) are the most easily removed, vanishing in a flash under the pulsed CO_2 laser beam. The treatment is somewhat painful, although the sensation lasts only for an instant. Patients describe the feeling as similar to a pop of sizzling bacon grease hitting the skin. Some people find it easily tolerable. Others require an anesthetic—either a topical numbing cream or an injection of lidocaine into the skin beneath the lesion.

Lased areas usually sting for a couple of hours afterwards. It can take anywhere from three to 10 days for the skin to rebuild a new surface over the treated spots. Lingering redness may persist for a couple of weeks up to several months. As sometimes happens when larger areas are lased, the treated spots may also start to turn brown (to hyperpigment) as they heal. If this happens, the doctor can prescribe a mild bleaching cream.

The most common benign superficial growths now commonly removed by laser vaporization are:

SKIN TAGS. The medical name for these harmless fleshy, usually minuscule, growths is acrochordons. Tiny collections of redundant epidermal cells that hang on fine stalks, they are rarely more than a fraction of an inch in size and may be flesh colored or any shade of brown. They most commonly appear in skin creases found on the eyelids or neck, under the breasts and arms and at the groin—often in groups. Skin tags rarely cause problems, although they can get irritated and may even bleed if they twist on their stalks or if they are rubbed by a piece of clothing such as a collar or bra strap.

The tendency to get skin tags appears to be inherited and affected by hormonal changes. Most common among people over 40 years old, they also frequently crop up during pregnancy, and in post-menopausal women and people with diabetes.

Skin tags are exceedingly easy to remove. The carbon dioxide laser vaporizes them instantly and the skin heals very quickly. The laser treatment's only drawback is its price. Some doctors charge more for using it and unless the growth is unusually large, other methods are just as effective. Tiny skin tags can be quickly burned off with an electric needle; the tag turns into a little charred scab that drops off in a few days, usually without a trace. They also may be frozen with liquid nitrogen or simply snipped off with scissors. Very large skin tags can be cut off and the base then cauterized with an electric needle —an effect similar to that of laser vaporization.

Once gone, a skin tag seldom returns in the same spot. But susceptible individuals usually grow new ones. Many people routinely go to their dermatologist every couple of years or so to have all the new tags removed.

SEBORRHEIC KERATOSES. People frequently confuse these common growths with warts. In fact they are little collections of the skin protein keratin, the substance that makes up the outer surface of the epidermis. Seborrheic keratoses usually start out as smooth, pale yellowish spots that turn into scaly tan, brown or gray plaques, sometimes with a slightly greasy feeling. They are typically raised above the surface of the skin, with sharp edges that make them look as if they have been applied from the outside. They are thought to be caused by age- or hormone-related changes to the keratinocytes, the cells that produce keratin.

Seborrheic keratoses may show up anywhere on the body, although they tend to be concentrated on the trunk. Sometimes they appear on the legs as grayish white growths that look like pieces of stucco, earning them the name "stucco keratoses." They range from a fraction of an inch in diameter to the size of a quarter or half dollar. They tend to multiply and to grow larger with time, some eventually developing into thick dark nodules.

Seborrheic keratoses are the most common benign skin

growths in America. Almost everybody past the age of 45 eventually gets a few of them; some people acquire hundreds. Sometimes they first appear in pregnancy. They are harmless in themselves, yet occasionally one will grow in such a way that its appearance mimics that of a skin cancer. In that case, the doctor may want to biopsy it before removing it. Seborrheic keratoses are usually easy to treat; they can be effectively removed with electrocautery or cryosurgery as well as a laser. But unless every last cell is eradicated, another keratosis will usually grow back in the same spot.

DERMATOSIS PAPULOSA NIGRA. This common benign condition, most frequently seen on people with dark skin tones, is a variant of seborrheic keratoses. The lesions are small, usually dome-shaped, dark brown or black bumps with a hard or warty texture. They are typically found on the cheeks, temples and neck.

Rarely seen in Caucasians, dermatosis papulosa nigra occurs in about 35 percent of all African-American adults. It can affect other dark-skinned ethnic groups such as Native Americans, Asians and Europeans of Mediterranean origin. Typically, it first appears in adolescence and the lesions increase in size and number with advancing age.

Because deeply pigmented skin is particularly vulnerable to skin darkening following an injury (post-inflammatory hyperpigmentation), any means of removing these lesions can leave a noticeable brown spot. Because of its precision, laser treatment is considered the least likely method to do so. If hyperpigmentation does occur, a mild bleaching cream will usually arrest the darkening quickly.

LINEAR EPIDERMAL NEVI. Although these growths are called nevi—the medical term for moles —they are not true moles. Rather they are the visible signs of a relatively rare congenital malformation of the skin which causes some epidermal cells to develop into scabby looking overgrowths. They usually appear at birth or shortly after as hard, horny, gray or brown bumps, often occurring in clusters. Individual lesions are pea-sized or larger, shaped in an irregular, roughly linear configuration.

Linear epidermal nevi were once regarded as all but untreatable. They are usually too large to be surgically excised without leaving a significant scar. And they typically grow back after being removed by more superficial methods, such as dermabrasion. Today, doctors regard resurfacing with the pulsed CO_2 laser as the treatment of choice for these lesions.

BENIGN DERMAL TUMORS

Dermal tumors are growths that can be found anywhere on the body and that reach into the skin's middle layer, the dermis. Because they are more deeply rooted, they are harder to remove than the more superficial epidermal tumors, and the process hurts more. Patients who have dermal tumors taken off without benefit of anesthesia describe the feeling as a much more intense and prolonged version of the hot bacon grease sensation. Even so, many people still find the transient discomfort of the laser more tolerable than the multiple injections of local anesthesia it sometimes takes to numb their skin before having these tumors removed. For those who do elect to have anesthesia, individual lesions are directly injected with small amounts of a local anesthetic such as lidocaine. For clusters of growths or very large lesions, the entire affected area of skin may be numbed with regional nerve blocks.

Benign dermal tumors vary greatly in size and severity, ranging from small and innocuous to extremely disfiguring. And they extend into the dermis at varying depths —some too deeply to be taken out entirely by any means, including the laser, without leaving some kind of mark—although the flat, faded spots that typically remain after laser treatment of dermal lesions is usually far less obvious than the scars produced by other means. Very often the most cosmetically desirable result comes from removing just enough of the abnormal tissue to flatten the area out, leaving the deepest part of the tumor behind. This way there is no scar and while the tumor may eventually reappear, it is likely to remain quiescent for years. If the growth does come back in the course of time, it can easily be removed again.

Some dermal tumors are subjected to multiple treatments with more than one type of laser. In these cases, the CO_2 laser is often used first to remove the bulky, more superficial portion of the growth and then a vascular- or pigment-specific laser zeros in on the underlying structures.

ANGIOFIBROMAS. Small firm nodules on the face, angiofibromas consist of strands of collagen-like fibers interlaced with tiny blood vessels. The lesions are dome-shaped, measuring from less than a sixteenth of an inch to a quarter of an inch in diameter. They are usually flesh-colored but may also be shades of red or brown; sometimes they develop a slightly warty texture.

These common growths typically show up for the first time when people are in their 30s through 50s. They are often mistaken for other things—including scars, moles or basal cell cancers. And they are sometimes a sign of underlying disease, so it is very important that they be carefully evaluated and perhaps subjected to a biopsy before they are removed with a laser.

Angiofibromas are usually leveled off with the CO_2 laser, which vaporizes the raised tissue. A small portion of the lesion does remain, but it usually cannot be detected once the area has healed, about four to six weeks later. If at that time, the remaining, deeper portion of the tumor can still be seen as a bit of reddish tissue, it may be treated with a vascular-specific laser. One to three treatments spaced about a month apart will lighten the lesion and further reduce its size by removing the tiny blood vessels that are adding bulk as well as causing redness.

NEUROFIBROMAS. Caused by an overgrowth of the fatty substance that surrounds nerve fibers in the skin, neurofibromas appear on the surface as soft, flesh colored papules. If you press on one, you can usually make it sink back at least partially into the skin. Neurofibromas are very common, cropping up on as many as ten percent of the general population. Appearing anywhere on the body, they are almost always very small and innocent. But they have the potential to grow extremely large and invasive. (The 19th century medical curiosity known as the "Elephant Man" was afflicted with neurofibromatosis, a rare condition that triggered wild, unrestrained growth of neurofibromas.)

A single treatment with the CO_2 laser can vaporize the raised portion of a neurofibroma and at least part of its dermal component. However, the laser usually cannot get to the bottom of the more deeply rooted of these lesions and thus those may eventually grow back. (Regrowth does not typically occur for many months or even years later.)

SEBACEOUS HYPERPLASIA. These small yellowish bumps, sometimes surrounding a central depression containing what looks like a large pore or blackhead, frequently develop on the cheeks, forehead and nose of people in their 40s or older. They represent the presence of enlarged oil glands under the skin. However, they do not produce oil and they do not cause an oily complexion. The bumps may look like small skin cancers and should be carefully examined, even subjected to a biopsy to rule out malignancy if the diagnosis is unclear. They typically increase in size and number over the years. Individual nodules can usually be completely removed in one session with the CO_2 laser, but susceptible individuals are likely to acquire new ones.

RHINOPHYMA. This is an extreme form of sebaceous hyperplasia that affects the oil glands in the skin on the nose. The condition, rarely seen in women, is common among older men with advanced cases of the skin-reddening vascular disorder, rosacea (Chapter 8, pages 142-144). The abnormally enlarged oil glands, and the excess oil inside them, thicken the skin and produce swollen lobes that may eventually enlarge the nose to twice its normal size or more.

It requires aggressive treatment with the CO_2 laser to treat rhinophyma. Multiple passes with the laser beam pare down the nodules by vaporizing the abnormal tissue. This can be very painful, so patients are usually anesthetized with local injections and appropriate nerve blocks prior to treatment.

Postoperative care for the nose is identical to that for any other laser-resurfaced area of the face (Chapter 2). Because rhinophyma is a condition that grows slowly over many years, it should not recur to any noticeable degree after laser resurfacing. If the underlying rosacea is still apparent after surgery, it can be treated with a vascular-specific laser (Chapter 8).

SYRINGOMAS. Benign tumors of the sweat glands, these tiny papules may crop up singly, or more typically in groups, anywhere on the face or chest, but are most common on the lower eyelids and upper cheeks. They have a pearly, translucent appearance and are usually flesh colored, although they may also be tan or brown.

The tendency to develop syringomas appears to be inherited. They first appear in early adulthood, and are more common among women than men. They may increase in size and sensitivity during pregnancy or when taking oral contraceptives.

Syringomas are persistent. They can be easily removed with the CO_2 laser, but may return within a couple of years or so.

XANTHELASMA. Associated with disturbances in cholesterol metabolism, xanthelasma appear as flat, yellow, irregularly shaped, cholesterol-filled plaques with a firm texture. Like syringomas, they frequently appear on the eyelids. They are difficult to remove, but can usually be improved and even eliminated with one or more CO_2 laser treatments.

DEEPER BENIGN TUMORS

Some benign growths that look similar to and may be confused with the dermal tumors listed above extend more deeply into the skin, down into the subcutis or fatty layer. They cannot be removed with a laser, but must be excised with a scalpel, usually leaving a small wound that requires one or more stitches to close. Two of the most common of these deeper benign tumors are:

SEBACEOUS CYSTS. These harmless growths consist of a cheesy material composed of keratin, oil gland secretions and other cellular debris contained in a small rigid walled sack. The entire globular mass must be surgically excised, or the cyst will grow back.

LIPOMAS, another type of benign skin tumor, result from over-production of fat cells inside the subcutis. The presence of a lipoma makes the skin bulge; if pressed, the area feels spongy. Excision or even liposuction can evacuate a lipoma.

MOLES

Moles, or nevi, as they are referred to medically, are small growths consisting of nevus cells, which are variants of melanocytes, the cells that produce the brown pigment melanin. Consequently, most moles contain an abundance of melanin, and therefore are most commonly treated with pigment-specific lasers which destroy brown cells, leaving the epidermis unscathed (see Chapter 5).

The exception are a group of moles called **benign compound nevi**. These are moles that have both an epidermal and a dermal component. They are generally raised because the proliferation of nevus cells pushes up the epidermis. They range in color from dark brown to flesh-colored.

Brown compound nevi can be removed with a pigment-specific laser, but the flesh-colored ones offer no melanin for those lasers to target. They are instead vaporized with a pulsed CO_2 laser in the same manner as the dermal tumors described above. As with other dermal lesions, the procedure may leave a small faded spot on the skin. Although there is always a chance that the mole will grow back, if it does not reappear within a year, it is likely gone for good.

Warts, or "verrucae," are benign tumors caused by a virus called the human papilloma virus (HPV). The visible part of a wart is an overgrowth of scaly epidermal cells. They can occur anywhere on the body, but are most frequently seen on the hands, feet, legs and genitals. Those that occur on the soles of the feet are known as plantar warts; those that develop around the nails are called periungual warts.

Warts respond unpredictably to any form of treatment. Conventional means of removal include burning them off with electric needles or acids (including the salicylic acid formulations found in over-the-counter wart patches and solutions) or freezing them with liquid nitrogen. Each of these methods destroys the viral-infected cells that constitute the visible portion of the wart. But the HPV virus can also be found in the skin as far away as half an inch from the center of the visible growth. These unseen, undestroyed viruses are what cause warts to recur and require re-treatment. Not only is this a nuisance, but repeatedly treating the same area can leave very obvious scars. Periungual warts, which are particularly difficult to reach and must be treated aggressively, may result in misshapen fingernails following treatment.

Warts that have resisted removal by other methods may be treated with two types of laser therapy. The pulsed CO_2 laser can vaporize large and multiple warts quickly, often completely obliterating them in a single session. Successful treatment generally involves vaporizing a large area, including what appears to be normal skin in order to get all of the wart virus. This is like a small skin resurfacing procedure; it is painful—usually requiring anesthesia —and there is a long healing period. There is also some danger of scarring if the wart is very deep and requires vaporization of a large area of tissue.

A less invasive way to lase away a wart is to attack the blood vessels that lie beneath the growth, feeding the virus that causes it. A vascular-specific laser can destroy those vessels, choking off the virus' blood supply and effectively starving it to death. This should get rid of the wart for good without leaving a scar. But it may be a long process, requiring as little as one or two treatments to as many as 10 or more spaced about a month apart.

Treatment with the vascular-specific laser is not as painful as with the CO_2 laser, but it hurts nonetheless. The repetitive pulsing of the laser beam on a single small site creates a significant amount of heat. Laser treatment of warts on the extremities is the most painful because those areas contain numerous small, sensitive nerve endings. Even so, most patients do not require anesthesia.

"It's like being jabbed with a hot electric needle. An incredibly focused sharp pain. And it has a cumulative effect," explained Jason, 37, who had been trying to get rid of recalcitrant warts on his fingers for two years.

"Afterward, it aches for the first hour or so, like a cut. But better this than all of the other things I've tried. This is far more desirable, even with the pain, because I think it's actually having some effect."

PRECANCEROUS SKIN GROWTHS

Precancerous skin growths are the result of abnormal cells that, for some reason, can no longer grow and reproduce in a normal fashion. No one understands the exact mechanism, but sun damage is certainly a major factor. Ultraviolet light damages the genetic material in skin cells. Instead of reproducing by creating new cells like themselves, they instead produce abnormal (or dysplastic) cells, which usually appear on the skin surface as a kind of scale—basically an increase in the horny material of the epidermis.

Precancerous growths are not dangerous in themselves. But they have the potential to progress to cancers, in which the abnormal cells start to proliferate wildly. The two common precancers listed here are considered good candidates for laser removal.

ACTINIC KERATOSES. The word actinic means sun-related, and these lesions (also called solar keratoses), are early signs of accumulated sun damage. They usually start to show up at about the time sun-induced wrinkles and brown spots first make their appearance. For most people this happens sometime during their mid-30s, although those whose work or recreation exposes them to excessive sun may see the effects of solar damage earlier. Fair-haired, fair-skinned individuals are the most susceptible. Actinic keratoses usually appear in groups on chronically sun-exposed areas such as the face, the scalp and the backs of the hands. Their location depends on an individual's sun exposure patterns. For example, a trucker who habitually drives with his left arm hanging out the window may have his left arm covered with pre-cancerous lesions while his right arm remains unmarked.

Actinic keratoses arise in the epidermis, initially appearing as smooth, flat red spots that do not go away. With time, the spots gradually get more irregular, scaly and rough. They may turn a darker red or reddish brown and acquire yellow or brown scales. Actinic keratoses usually can easily be diagnosed on sight, but it sometimes takes a biopsy to tell for sure. They sometimes look like seborrheic keratoses, although they are not so well defined and tend to be more pinkish in color. Sometimes they shed spontaneously, leaving a red, inflamed, depressed base out of which grows another keratosis.

Because actinic keratoses may progress to squamous cell skin cancer, doctors consider it important to treat them. They are commonly removed by freezing the affected areas with liquid nitrogen (cryosurgery) or though the application of a chemical called 5-fluorouracil (Efudex), which seeks out and destroys precancerous cells.

Actinic keratoses can easily be removed with the pulsed CO_2 laser. The treatment is the same as for benign epidermal growths: the laser quickly vaporizes the abnormal tissues causing brief, transitory pain. The skin may be numbed first with a topical anesthetic, or injection with lidocaine. Isolated lesions are usually vaporized individually. If there are numerous lesions, as is often the case on the face or scalp, the entire area may be resurfaced with the laser or with cryosurgery. Full facial resurfacing has the advantage of removing precancerous cells that may not yet be apparent to the naked eye.

ACTINIC CHELITIS. This is another condition caused by overexposure to the sun. It is characterized by chronically inflamed and scaly lips. It is very common among people who spend much of their lives outdoors. The affected lip mucous membrane becomes chronically chapped and eroded, bleeding easily.

Resurfacing the lips with a pulsed CO_2 laser is now considered the treatment of choice for actinic chelitis. It usually takes two to three passes with the laser to vaporize the abnormal tissue. This is very painful, so the mouth is usually injected with nerve blocking medication beforehand. Afterwards, the lips hurt and appear raw and swollen, making it difficult to talk or eat for several days. Fortunately, the mouth heals rapidly, and the treated lips feel and appear close to normal within a week or two.

SKIN CANCERS

Cancerous skin tumors are caused by the unrestrained growth of abnormal cells. They may expand locally, growing into adjacent areas. Or, in their most dangerous form, they can spread systemically by the process known as metastasis, in which malignant cells migrate through the body via the bloodstream or lymph system. There are three forms of skin cancer, only one of which is generally considered a suitable candidate for removal by laser.

BASAL CELL CANCER. Basal cell cancer is the most common form of skin cancer. It usually occurs on sun-exposed areas of skin. The lesions appear as raised, somewhat translucent or pearly bumps. They may ulcerate, bleed and crust. People sometimes mistake the bumps for pimples and try to squeeze them or scratch them away.

Basal cell cancers rarely metastasize so they are not usually considered life-threatening. However, they can grow to huge sizes, causing extensive damage to adjacent normal skin and to underlying structures. Ulcerated lesions bleed and may become infected.

After confirming the diagnosis of basal cell cancer by biopsy, a surgeon can evaporate the growths with a pulsed CO_2 laser. The skin is usually numbed with anesthetic injected under the affected area and the cancerous tissue is vaporized with several passes of the laser beam, usually also removing an extra amount of normal skin around the border.

Once the cancerous growth has been removed, the doctor

will want to see you at least yearly for a skin check. Sometimes a lesion will grow back. If that happens, it should not be treated with the laser again, but excised surgically so that the tissue can be carefully examined in a laboratory.

SQUAMOUS CELL CARCINOMA. The second most common form of skin cancer, squamous cell cancer, appears as elevated opaque pink bumps or warty, mushroom-like growths. They commonly occur on the rim of the ears, the face, lips and hands, often in chronically sun-exposed sites. The lesions are more frequent on areas of skin that have been subjected to severe burns or radiation. Squamous cell cancers tend to ulcerate and bleed, and they may become infected. As a rule, those caused by sun damage seldom metastasize. But others may, so biopsy confirmation is very important. Squamous cell cancers are not generally considered suitable candidates for laser surgery. Instead, doctors usually excise them surgically.

MALIGNANT MELANOMA. This is the least common and most serious form of skin cancer. It is potentially fatal; over 6,000 people in the U.S. die each year from malignant melanoma. Anyone can develop it, although some people are regarded as being at particularly high risk: individuals with fair skin who sunburn easily and tan poorly (Phototypes I and II); people who have a large number of unusually shaped moles or freckles on their bodies; those with a family history of melanoma and anyone who has had a severe sunburn during childhood.

The lesions may first appear as abnormal looking moles or pigmented spots. Common danger signs include asymmetry, in which one half of the mole appears different from the other half; a mole that is variegated in color or has irregular scalloped or indistinct borders; or a mole that is larger than 7 mm in diameter—about the size of a pencil eraser. Anyone who has any of these signs should consult a doctor immediately. Malignant melanomas metastasize quickly, spreading cancerous cells through the body.

A malignant melanoma should never, under any circumstances, be removed with a laser. The only acceptable treatment is what is known as wide excision—surgically cutting out the lesion and the surrounding skin and underlying tissue in order to ensure that all the cancerous cells have been removed. Patients may also be treated with a course of radiation or chemotherapy.

SKIN CARE AFTER LASER REMOVAL OF SKIN GROWTHS

Laser removal of superficial skin growths leaves small wounds that usually heal very quickly. For the first few days, the areas may ooze, crust and be somewhat swollen and tender. It will take three to 10 days for the skin to rebuild a new surface over the treated spots.

1. Keep the treated areas covered with an antibiotic ointment such as bacitracin while there is any oozing or crusting.

2. If the treated areas swell, apply ice packs. If crusts form, apply wet compresses to soak and dissolve them; do not try to pick them off.

3. You can apply makeup to the treated areas as soon as the scabs have cleared. Be very careful when removing your makeup; rubbing hard will retard healing and can lead to permanent changes in your skin's texture.

4. If you are going outside, be sure to liberally apply a sunscreen of SPF 15 or greater to the treated areas. They will be abnormally sensitive to the sun as long as they appear red. Sun exposure could cause permanent changes in skin color or texture at this stage.

5. The spots may remain pink for several weeks or months. And, as sometimes happens when larger areas are lased, the treated spots may also begin to turn brown (to hyperpigment) as they heal. If this happens, inform your doctor so that an appropriate mild bleaching cream can be prescribed.

CHAPTER FIVE

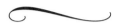

TARGETING MELANIN:
FRECKLES, AGE SPOTS, MOLES
AND OTHER BROWN PATCHES

*G*etting rid of almost any brown-colored spot or patch on the skin—whether it is a mole, a freckle, an age spot or a brown birthmark—is one of the trickiest problems in cosmetic dermatology. Until the most recent advances in laser surgery, most of these brown lesions could not be removed at all without leaving another discolored patch or a scar. And even today with the latest technology, many of these spots and splotches still stubbornly resist all attempts to dislodge them.

It is not uncommon for brown lesions that have been removed by a laser to come back—sometimes within weeks, other times after many months. Certain ones may even appear darker than they were before they were treated, apparently because the laser stimulates the skin to step up its production of the pigment melanin. In other cases, brown spots seem to almost completely resist the laser, only imperceptibly lightening despite repeated treatments. On the other hand, some patients see treated areas of skin lighten immediately and continue to lighten steadily for months afterwards. These reactions are highly individual and it is virtually impossible to know ahead of time how any given patient will respond to laser treatment for a pigmented lesion.

Given this, it is no wonder that people who have been treated for brown pigmented lesions represent a broad spectrum of patient satisfaction. It takes multiple laser treatments to remove most brown spots, and people who have undergone repeated surgery only to see little or no improvement in their skin are understandably disappointed. Some are irate. "I'm not sure I see the point any more," said one woman who went through five laser treatments to remove two moles. "I can see they're a little lighter. But they're still there. I could go on for months to get to where you can't see them anymore. It would cost a lot of money. My insurance won't pay for it. And after all that, they might even come back. Why bother?" Another woman, treated just one time for brown age spots, never returned for a second laser session, complaining that the long healing period made her look awful, and afterwards she could not see any difference in her skin.

On the other hand, people for whom the laser works are often thrilled by the eventual results. Eve, at 40, had never owned a bathing suit, a pair or shorts or a short skirt because of crippling embarrassment over a café-au-lait birthmark just below the calf on her left leg. "It caused me so much emotional trauma all of my life. I was unmercifully teased as a child and by the time I grew up, I wanted that thing gone so much I was willing to cut my leg off."

Over a period of 12 months, Eve underwent five laser treatments which finally rid her of her birthmark. She was elated. "It was like a miracle," she exclaimed. "About five months after the last treatment, the mark seemed to vanish overnight.

It completely changed my life. I can take my children to the pool. I can wear nice clothes. I've made a pact with myself that I will never own another dress below my knees."

Michelle was seemingly covered with moles. She had been born with some of them, others had appeared over the years, especially during her 20s when her torso, arms and legs became thickly dotted with hundreds of dark brown spots. "I saw doctors who scared me half to death with warnings about cancer, but when I had some of the larger moles removed surgically, there wasn't anything wrong with them. They just looked bad."

This strikingly lovely young woman, who had been a professional model, grew miserably self-conscious about her appearance. "All I wanted to do was cover up. I didn't want to wear anything that revealed my skin. And I didn't think there was anything I could do about it. The moles I had taken off left big white scars. I thought I was stuck with the others."

It didn't seem at first that laser surgery would be the answer either. "It took forever. I think I had more than 12 treatments— I lost count. But now that it's over, I'm happy because my skin looks beautiful. My mother can't believe it. There are still some moles, but in most places it looks like I never had any at all. "

Using Lasers on Brown Spots

Everything that shows up as brown on the skin—whether it is a freckle, an age spot, a brown birthmark or a summer tan— is in some way a manifestation of the highly complex human pigmentary system. Melanocytes, the specialized cells that produce the skin pigment melanin, arise in the lowest (or basal) layer of the epidermis. They synthesize melanin granules inside microscopic packages called melanosomes. As melanocytes

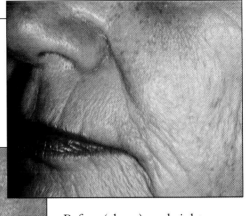

he left cheek of a
-year-old woman with
rinkles caused by excessive
n exposure (solar rhytides).

Before (above), and eight
weeks after (left) resurfacing
with the high-energy pulsed
carbon dioxide laser.
(Chap 2)

54-year-old
man with deep
inkles around the
uth. Before (above,
ht) and three weeks
er (below, right)
urfacing with the
h-energy pulsed
bon dioxide laser.
e very smooth texture
the skin is caused by
idual swelling; as it
olves, some of the
inkles may recur.
hap 2)

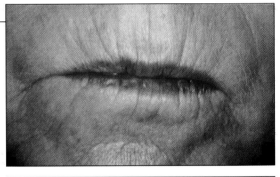

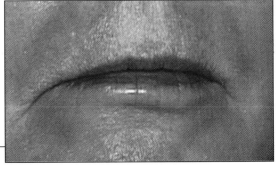

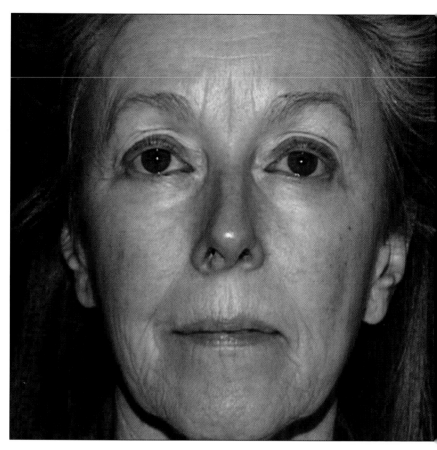

Before (above) and
four weeks after full
face (opposite, top)
resurfacing with the
high-energy pulsed
carbon dioxide laser.
The almost glassy
texture of the skin
and the distinct pink
color are typical at
this stage. (Chap 2)

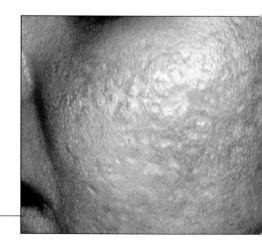

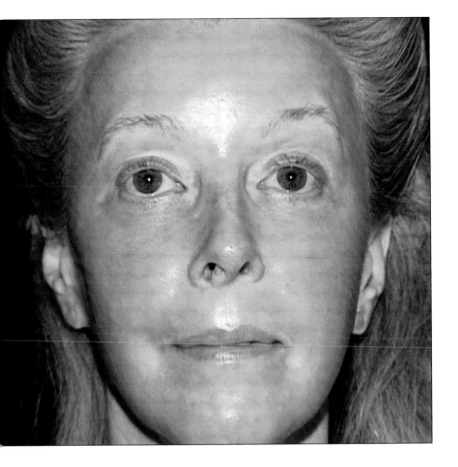

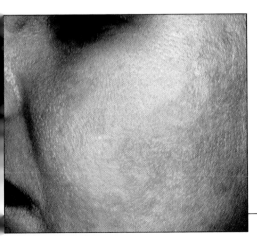

The left cheek of a 32-year-old woman with depressed (atrophic) acne scars. Before (opposite, below) and eight months after (left) resurfacing with the high-energy pulsed carbon dioxide laser. (Chap 3)

A 24-year-old woman with a professional tattoo on the left ankle. Before (right) and six months after (below) the final of nine treatments (over the course of two years) with

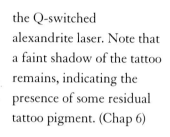

the Q-switched alexandrite laser. Note that a faint shadow of the tattoo remains, indicating the presence of some residual tattoo pigment. (Chap 6)

A 53-year-old woman with rosacea. Before (right) and three months after (opposite, right) the last of four treatments with the 585nm pulsed dye laser. (Chap 8)

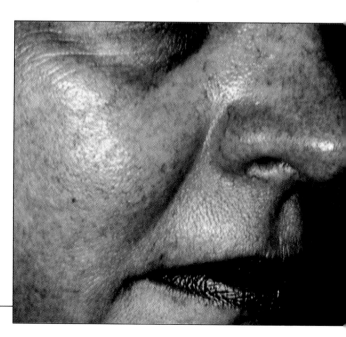

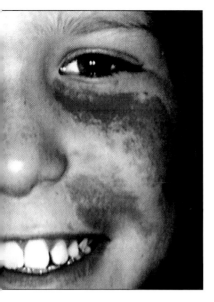 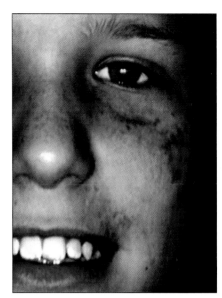

An 11-year-old girl with a port-wine stain on the left side of her face. Before (above, left) and six months after (above, right) the eighth treatment (over the course of two years) with the 585nm pulsed dye laser. (Chap 7)

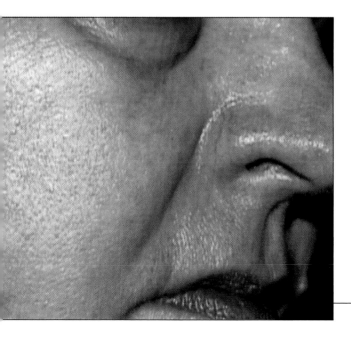

A 61-year-old woman with poikiloderma caused by excessive sun exposure on the left side of her neck.

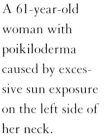

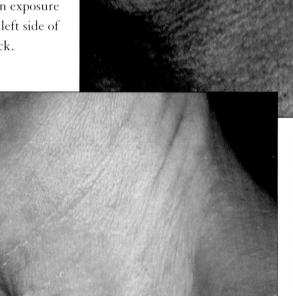

Before (above) and five months after (left) the third of three treatments with the 585nm pulsed dye laser. (Chap 8)

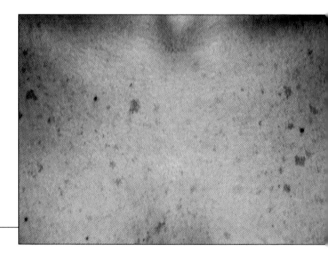

A 33-year-old woman with one-year-old post-pregnancy abdominal stretch marks.

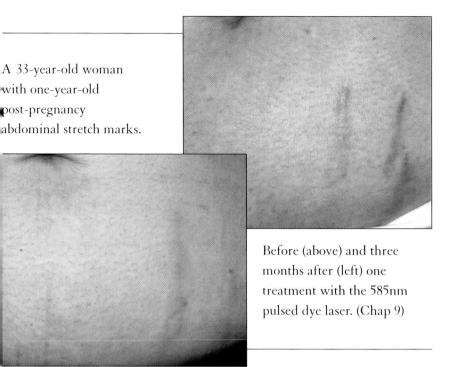

Before (above) and three months after (left) one treatment with the 585nm pulsed dye laser. (Chap 9)

A 40-year-old woman with extensive "age spots" (solar lentigines) caused by sun damage on her chest. Before (opposite, below) and seven weeks after (below) the second of two treatments with the 510nm pigmented lesion pulsed dye laser. (Chap 5)

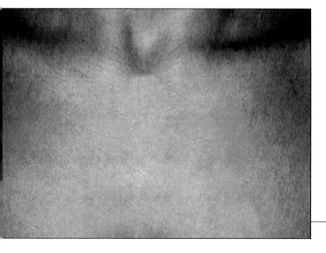

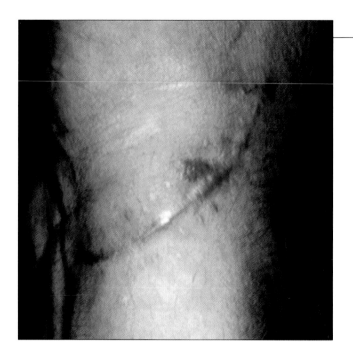

A 16-year-old boy with a raised red traumatic scar on the inside of his left arm. Before (above) and three and a half months after (right) the last of three treatments with the 585nm pulsed dye laser. (Chap 9)

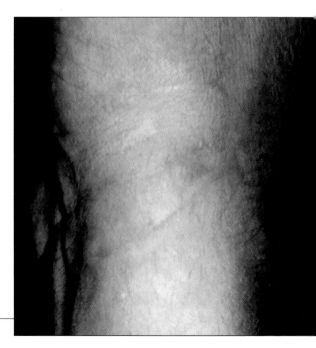

migrate to the surface of the epidermis, they transfer the melanin-laden melanosomes to other skin cells and to the hair follicles. This is what gives people their individual skin and hair color.

Almost all of the abnormal brown patches and spots that people acquire result from some change or malfunction in this process of pigment production and transfer. Such changes can be triggered—or may be influenced—by a number of factors. Exposure to the sun, hormonal activity and drugs can all either stimulate or inhibit melanin synthesis. These factors may also affect the transfer of melanosomes to keratinocytes. Or the entire mechanism can be altered by elements in a person's diet or changes in metabolism.

Most of the lasers that are now used to eradicate brown lesions work by targeting melanin through the action of selective photothermolysis. This means that the laser is tuned to emit a wavelength that is absorbed only by melanin granules. The laser's beam penetrates the skin and zeros in on the melanin contained in different cells. The melanin absorbs the light wave, heats up and destroys the surrounding melanosome.

A number of lasers have been specifically designed to selectively eliminate pigmented tissue in this fashion. The safest and most effective in use today employ a rapid-fire shuttering system called Q-switching that flashes the laser beam on and off in nanosecond bursts to ensure that destructive heat does not build up and burn the skin or damage its collagen structure, leaving a scar. However, the laser beam is so powerful that when it hits melanin-containing cells, they literally explode, and this does cause some damage to surrounding tissues. The result is usually a small bruise or red spot, and sometimes a minor wound that breaks the skin. These small injuries typically clear up within a couple of weeks without scarring.

The three most common Q-switched lasers are the ruby laser, the neodymium: yttrium aluminum garnet (Nd:YAG) and the alexandrite laser. In each, the laser beam passes though the named crystal, which determines the powerful light's precise characteristics. Brown lesions are also frequently treated with a laser called the Pigmented Lesion Dye Laser (PLDL), in which the electronically-pulsed beam passes through a chamber filled with a green-colored dye.

All of these lasers are extremely effective in destroying melanin. Unfortunately, the final visible result that any of them produces can vary widely. Even though melanin itself is an easy target to hit, the pigmentary system is so complex and so likely to be influenced by other agents that doctors cannot always foresee or control all the ways in which a laser may affect it. Darkly pigmented skin is particularly unpredictable and difficult to treat because its more naturally abundant melanin filters the laser light and influences its effects on the target cells.

Many patients will experience some temporary skin lightening (transient hypopigmentation) over the treated areas. This is because a certain amount of normal melanin is destroyed by the laser along with the more abundant melanin contained in the target lesions. But unlike the far more serious condition known as permanent hypopigmentation, which results from destruction of the pigment-producing apparatus, transient hypopigmentation is temporary. The skin typically regains its normal color in one to three months.

The key to permanently removing any brown lesion seems to lie in removing every last trace of abnormal brown pigment—no matter how many treatments it takes. Although doctors have no idea why this occurs, it appears that once all of the pigment containing melanosomes in any given lesion are eradicated, the pigment-producing cells in that area often get the message to stop overproducing melanin. Unfortunately, it sometimes proves impossible to totally eradicate all abnormal brown pigment in some patients.

Today, clinical and laboratory researchers are actively exploring ways to better the odds in making laser treatment of pigmented lesions more accurate and predictable. In the meanwhile, patients should be aware that getting rid of any brown lesion can be very much a hit-or-miss proposition. Some clear up beautifully; others barely budge. So it is extremely important to be carefully evaluated and treated by a dermatologist who has extensive experience in treating brown pigment with lasers. Bear in mind that the most experienced laser surgeons are likely to be the ones expressing the most reservations when predicting the outcome of treatment.

EPIDERMAL PIGMENTED LESIONS

Three types of superficial brown spots (or macules) confined entirely to the epidermis, are among the most common of the brown lesions being removed by lasers today.

FRECKLES. The familiar freckle is a small brown spot that shows up on the exposed skin of very fair-skinned, fair-haired people as a protective response to solar radiation. People are born with the tendency to freckle, although no one is actually born with freckles. The spots usually appear in early childhood, after a youngster has been exposed to the sun. The ultraviolet light seems to stimulate some melanocytes to grow larger and become more active in producing melanin and transferring it to keratinocytes. The pigmented keratinocytes group together in little clusters that appear on the surface as light brown spots. The medical name for them is ephelides.

Traditionally, Americans have long judged a freckled face to be endearing, particularly on a youngster. But some adults consider their own generous sprinkling of freckles too generous or downright unattractive and are eager to have them removed.

LENTIGINES. This is the collective term for a group of very common lesions that take their name from the term lentigo. They resemble lentils in that they are small, brown and round or oval in shape. They generally start out only a few millimeters in diameter, but can enlarge to several centimeters.

There are many forms of lentigo. Some of them may be associated with underlying health problems, but the type that concerns most people, the solar lentigo (or lentigo senilis) is the product of accumulated sun damage. This is the dreaded "age spot" or "liver spot" that most frequently appears on customarily exposed areas of skin, especially the face, the scalp, the backs of the hands and the arms. Solar lentigines increase in number and size with age, usually in proportion to the amount of sunlight a person has been subjected to over the years.

Solar lentigines do not turn into skin cancers. However, they should be carefully evaluated by a dermatologist before they are removed, because in appearance they may closely resemble a malignant lesion called Hutchinson's melanotic freckle or lentigo maligna. This is a sun-induced malignant melanoma that typically appears on the face, forearms or trunk. It evolves slowly over many years, gradually spreading out into a large, unevenly pigmented stain. This is a dangerous form of skin cancer that must be surgically excised; it should not be treated with a laser.

Freckles and age spots can often be successfully lightened in several ways that are simpler and more cost-effective than using a laser. One of the most common is cryosurgery—

freezing the lesions with liquid nitrogen. Doctors also advise treating superficial brown spots by avoiding the sun, using a strong sunscreen and applying skin fading creams containing a melanin-inhibiting agent such as hydroquinone. These steps can considerably minimize the appearance of brown patches, although it takes persistence and time—at least four to six months—to see significant fading.

Laser surgeons employ several laser techniques to eradicate freckles and age-spots. One involves the same pulsed CO_2 laser used for resurfacing. In many cases, the spots come off in the course of a full-face resurfacing operation. The melanin-containing cells are vaporized along with all of the other epidermal cells. The skin then builds itself a new surface without the brown patches.

However, it is too dangerous to use the CO_2 laser on the scar-prone chest, hands and arms, where many people have prominent brown discolorations. Laser surgeons remove these lesions—and other isolated ones on the face, scalp or elsewhere—with one of the pigment-specific Q-switched lasers or a green light laser such as the pigmented lesion dye laser (PLDL). Treatment with any one of these lasers is far less painful than having the epidermis removed with the resurfacing laser. Patients describe the feeling as similar to that of having a rubber band snapped against the skin. Because the pain only lasts for a brief instant, most people are treated without anesthesia; patients who find the sensation too uncomfortable are given a local anesthetic.

More than one treatment is usually necessary in order to get rid of all traces of brown. Two or three laser sessions spaced about six weeks apart are typical. And there is no guarantee that any individual lesion may not come back some day. It almost certainly will recur if the patient does not subsequently shun the sun. Otherwise, complications are rare. Some patients experience temporary skin lightening; others may notice superficial changes in skin texture.

CAFÉ-AU-LAIT SPOTS. Like freckles or lentigines, these large, pale brown patches are comprised of melanin-containing cells confined entirely to the epidermis. The spots may be associated with any one of several relatively rare diseases. However, most are birthmarks that occur for no known reason in up to 10 percent of the normal population. People are born with macules on their skin that may only gradually become visible as a person passes through childhood or becomes exposed to the sun. They appear as light tan to pale brown spots with sharply defined borders, ranging from less than an inch to about eight inches in diameter. They do not go away on their own.

Café-au-lait spots should be carefully examined to determine if they result from any disease. Otherwise, the lesions are not considered dangerous because they have a very low potential to turn malignant. Because of their size, however, they can be very disfiguring.

Café-au-lait macules are comprised of abnormal, often unusually large melanosomes. They are extremely difficult to eradicate. A physician may have to administer as many as 10 or more treatments spaced at 2-month intervals to rid a patient of all the pigment-containing cells. About 15 percent of patients experience some temporary skin lightening (transient hypopigmentation) afterwards.

As with freckles and lentigines, it is extremely important to eliminate all of the visible brown pigment. If even a few of the abnormal melanin-containing cells are left to linger in the skin, they will stimulate the growth of a new macule. If this occurs, it will likely happen within a year after laser treatment.

DERMAL PIGMENTED LESIONS

Some pigmented lesions are composed of melanin-containing cells lodged in the skin's middle layer, or dermis. Before the advent of pigment-specific lasers, these marks could not be removed by any means without leaving a very noticeable scar. Today they are effectively treated with any of the Q-switched laser systems.

The procedure is virtually the same as for epidermal lesions, although because the laser must penetrate more deeply in order to reach the pigmented areas, it must be adjusted to a slightly higher energy level. This creates more heat which tends to make treatments more painful. Side effects include temporary skin lightening (hypopigmentation) or darkening (post-inflammatory hyperpigmentation) within the lased areas.

Multiple treatments, from four to eight or more, are typically necessary to clear up a dermal pigmented lesion. Treatments are spaced at eight to 12 week intervals to allow the skin to heal. The lased area usually appears dramatically lighter after the first session. Subsequent treatments show increasingly less reaction to the laser as the amount of pigment in the skin decreases. To help compensate for this falling-off effect, doctors may have to increase the laser's power a small amount at each subsequent session causing a proportionate increase in patient discomfort.

As with epidermal pigmented lesions, the result of laser therapy is unpredictable. Some lesions clear up entirely, others not at all. Those that only partially lighten after multiple treatments usually will darken or recur within one year

Three dermal pigmented lesions are now routinely treated by laser:

BLUE NEVUS. A blue nevus is a benign tumor composed of melanocytes in the dermis. It shows up on the surface as a raised papule, up to about one-third inch in diameter. Even though it is comprised of a brown pigment (melanin), it usually appears to the eye as a deep blue or black shade that results from the manner in which the overlying skin scatters the light. Blue nevi are most common on darker skin tones, usually appearing spontaneously on children or young adults, although the lesions can also be present at birth or appear in the elderly.

NEVUS OF OTA. Nevus of Ota consists of multiple small, dark, bluish-gray spots that coalesce to form a patch. It is usually located on one side of the face around the eye, cheek and temple, giving the appearance of a blackened eye. It most commonly occurs in patients with darker skin types, particularly among people of Asian ancestry.

NEVUS OF ITO. A rare skin condition closely related to nevus of Ota, nevus of Ito is a bluish-gray discoloration, usually located on a shoulder or upper arm. It is almost exclusively seen among people of Japanese ancestry.

COMBINED EPIDERMAL AND DERMAL PIGMENTED LESIONS

Of all the common pigmentary disorders, the most stubborn and unpredictable to treat are those with a combination of epidermal and dermal pigment. Unfortunately, this category includes two of the more common of the brown lesions that patients wish to have removed for cosmetic reasons: post-inflammatory hyperpigmentation and melasma, "the mask of pregnancy." A third, more rare combination lesion, called Becker's nevus, can be equally difficult to eradicate.

The use of lasers to treat these lesions is still very much a matter of investigation. In all three cases, lasers offer a treatment option that may or may not prove effective in clearing up the brown areas. So it is truly best to consult a laser surgeon with extensive experience in the field.

POST-INFLAMMATORY HYPERPIGMENTATION. Any time the skin is injured or inflamed, it may turn perceptibly darker or hyperpigmented. This can occur in small localized areas, as often happens following an injury. Or the darkening may be diffuse and widespread, usually as a result of excessive sun exposure. The latter may be particularly severe on areas of skin that have been sensitized by any one of a number of photosensitizing substances contained in many drugs and cosmetics. Some women, for example, develop hyperpigmented patches where they customarily spray perfume or cologne.

In many instances, the dark areas come from excess pigment that is confined entirely to the epidermis. This epidermal hyperpigmentation is the result of the skin stepping up its production of melanin in order to protect itself from further injury. The most common example of epidermal hyperpigmentation is a suntan. Another example is the darkening that frequently occurs during the healing period following laser resurfacing.

Epidermal post-inflammatory hyperpigmention is usually a transient condition; the overproduction of melanin is a temporary response to a specific trauma. If the skin is allowed to heal without further injury, the melanocytes eventually stop overproducing melanin and the skin gradually returns to its normal color. The brown patches will persist, however, if the skin is re-injured or exposed to ultraviolet light. Either event will stimulate the skin to produce more melanin and thus maintain the brown stain.

Conversely, simply protecting the skin and avoiding the sun may be all it takes to clear the spot up. The lightening process can be improved upon with skin fading creams and light peels, as described on pages 50–51 (Dark Skin and Post-Surgical Skin Darkening).

Hyperpigmentation with a dermal component—in which dark pigment settles in the dermis—is far more difficult to treat. No one really understands the exact mechanism behind it. Inflammation may cause some degeneration in the basal cell layer of the epidermis, allowing melanosomes to drop into the underlying dermis where they become lodged inside capsule-like entities called macrophages. In some cases, dermal darkening is not related to melanin at all, but instead marks the presence of hemosiderin, a yellowish-brown pigment produced by the breakdown of red blood cells following an injury.

As with epidermal hyperpigmentation, dermal hyperpigmentation tends to occur more commonly and more severely among people with naturally dark skin. Curiously, the seriousness of the injury or degree of inflammation seems to have little influence on how deeply the skin becomes hyperpigmented; traumas as mild as an insect bite sometimes produce very dark patches, while serious injuries may produce scars that show no darkening at all. Or vice versa. Again, no one can really say why.

Whatever the exact cause, most dermatologists treat dermal hyperpigmentation cautiously. The key element is scrupulous avoidance of the sun—by staying in the shade, wearing protective clothing and liberally applying a broad-spectrum sunscreen containing chemical agents that block both UVA and UVB radiation. Skin fading creams containing hydroquinone—sometimes combined with retinoic acid (Retin-A) and glycolic acid to gently peel the skin, or corticosteroids to decrease inflammation—can also help lighten the brown marks.

The results of laser treatment have so far been mixed. Doctors using both pulsed dye and various Q-switched lasers have reported results ranging from complete clearance after a couple of treatments to virtually no change at all despite multiple treatments.

MELASMA. The so-called "mask of pregnancy" is a form of hyperpigmentation associated with hormonal activity. It occurs to some extent in 50 to 70 percent of all pregnant women, usually appearing in the second and third trimesters, and almost always gradually fading away within a year following delivery. Melasma is also common among women who take oral contraceptives.

Melasma results from an overproduction of melanin. It appears as a symmetrical light to dark brown area on the face, particularly the cheeks. Like other forms of hyperpigmentation, the excess pigment can occur solely in the epidermis or it may extend into the dermis below. Generally, epidermal melasma has very sharp borders. Melasma that is principally dermal has a hazier appearance because the pigment lies deeper in the skin and overlying layers of skin blur its outlines.

Epidermal melasma tends to fade well on its own; dermal melasma is more stubborn and long-lasting. In either case, the brown areas can usually be lessened by avoiding the sun, applying fading creams and, in some cases, treating the dark areas with superficial chemical peels.

So far, the experience in treating melasma with lasers has been extremely disappointing. Doctors have tried a number of lasers on the lesions. In many cases, the lasers have had little or no effect. In other instances, patients have seen immediate clearing of the brown areas, followed within weeks by complete recurrence. Frequently, the repigmented areas appear darker than they were originally.

BECKER'S NEVUS. Although called a nevus, the medical term for mole, this large, irregularly-shaped brown lesion is actually a superficial tumor that arises from abnormal development of epidermal and dermal cells. It is most commonly seen in adolescent boys, usually appearing as a tan, textured stain extensive enough to spread over one shoulder or all the way across the back. Typically, it contains a number of coarse hairs.

Possibly triggered by hormonal changes associated with puberty, Becker's nevi tend to run in families. They are benign and once in place, they remain for life without changing significantly in appearance.

Because of their large size and the fact that there is no medical reason to remove them, most doctors leave Becker's nevi in place. Laser surgery, the only practical way to remove them without scarring, has shown only mixed success. Some doctors have removed the lesions entirely in two to six sessions with a ruby or pulsed dye laser. Others have been able to achieve only partial clearing despite multiple treatments. In some instances, laser treatment has caused Becker's nevi to turn an ashy gray color.

MOLES

The medical term for a mole is nevus and the cells that comprise it are called nevus cells. Nevus cells are a variation of melanocytes and, like melanocytes, they synthesize melanin. However, they cannot transfer the brown pigment to other skin cells.

Nevus cells clump together in a number of different

configurations and they appear at various depths in the skin. These differences account for the great variation in the appearance of different moles. They are broadly divided into two groups, congenital and acquired. The latter are further separated into three sub-categories depending on where the nevus cells appear in the skin.

Using lasers to remove moles is a subject of controversy in the medical community. Whether it is vaporized with a pulsed CO_2 laser (as are the benign compound nevi described in Chapter 4) or subjected to a pigment-specific laser that selectively destroys the melanin-containing nevus cells, a laser-eradicated mole is destroyed in place. This leaves no tissue available for laboratory examination, which is the conventional fate of any surgically-excised mole.

Moreover, people who are born with congenital moles or who have a large number of acquired moles are statistically more at risk for developing a malignant melanoma, the most dangerous form of skin cancer. An estimated 18 percent of congenital moles, usually the very large, irregularly-shaped ones, may eventually become cancerous; between one and five percent of small congenital moles may become malignant. In people with abundant acquired moles, melanoma usually forms independently; the existing moles rarely turn malignant themselves. However, a long-standing mole will sometimes rarely and mysteriously undergo a change that proves cancerous.

The unpredictable nature of even the most seemingly innocent moles has led to two schools of thought on laser treatment of moles. Some doctors believe that since the laser reduces the overall amount of pigment in a given mole, this lessens the chance of it ever altering in a dangerous manner. Other doctors feel that once the pigment is removed by laser treatment, it may prove difficult or impossible to detect the development of malignant change.

There have been no documented cases of cancers developing in moles that have been laser irradiated. And at the present time, the general consensus is that it is safe to use a laser on small (roughly 1/4 inch or less in diameter), long-standing moles. The best candidates are moles that are flat or nearly flat, and circular or nearly circular, with smooth borders and a uniform color.

Moles that fit those criteria may be found among any of those described below.

CONGENITAL MOLES (Congenital Melanocytic Nevi). These are moles that are present on an infant at birth. They are relatively uncommon, occurring in only about one percent of newborns; children who are born with them rarely have more than one. Most of the lesions are less than one-quarter inch across, although they may be so large that they cover large parts of the body—the entire back, for example.

Congenital moles are usually dark brown in color and display dark, prominent hairs. As a child ages, the mole may deepen even more in color and become elevated. Large congenital moles tend to extend deep into the dermis, smaller ones are more superficial.

Because large (or giant) congenital moles carry a relatively high lifetime risk for turning malignant, some pediatricians recommend that they be removed from young children as a protective measure. Small and medium-sized lesions usually can be easily excised. A very large congenital mole can only be removed though a major surgical procedure that usually involves multiple operations and skin grafting.

Laser removal of congenital moles may eventually prove to be a promising alternative. But it remains experimental. So far, a few doctors have attempted it in controlled studies and the results have been mixed. Usually the lesions clear up only partially and they frequently recur.

ACQUIRED MOLES (Acquired Melanocytic Nevi). These are the common moles that appear spontaneously from childhood through middle age, typically peaking at ages two to three, at puberty and again between 11 and 18. Most people do not acquire new moles after the age of 50. There are three classes of acquired melanocytic nevi.

JUNCTIONAL NEVI. All of the nevus cells are contained in the epidermis. The moles are usually light tan to very dark brown, hairless and smooth, although some may be slightly raised. They range from pinpoint size to about 1 cm in diameter. This is the common mole that appears on children and adolescents; additional ones may appear at any age, although rarely after a person is in his or her 50s. They frequently darken with pregnancy or hormonal changes. The tendency to develop these moles appears to be genetic, and in some families, they appear at similar sites on the body for generation after generation.

A pigment-specific laser is used to remove these moles. Just as when used on other brown lesions, the laser beam targets melanin—-in this instance, the melanin contained in the nevus cells. Treatments are delivered every one or two months until the desired degree of lightening has occurred.

COMPOUND NEVI. These are usually raised, smooth bordered moles composed of nevus cells in the epidermis and dermis. They range in texture from very smooth to extremely nodular or warty to the touch. They often contain hair. They are typically uniform in color, ranging from all shades of brown and tan to flesh-colored.

INTRADERMAL NEVI. Composed of nevus cells contained entirely in the dermis, these moles are uniformly colored shades of tan or brown and are usually dome-shaped from the pressure of clumped nevus cells pushing up the skin's surface.

Except for flesh-colored compound nevi, which are removed with the pulsed CO_2 laser (Chapter 4), both compound and intradermal nevi can be treated with any one of the pigment-specific lasers.

The procedure is the same as for other pigmented dermal lesions. It usually takes several treatments at six to 10-week intervals to completely remove a mole. This varies greatly among patients, and may even be different for different moles on the same person.

The long-term prognosis for laser-eradicated moles is about the same as for other pigmented lesions. In general, if any melanin in a given mole is left behind, the mole is likely to return some day. If, however, all the melanin is eliminated, that area of the skin may stop producing new nevus cells. As a rule of thumb, a mole that does not reappear within a year is probably gone for good.

DANGEROUS MOLES

Although doctors regard all moles with a certain degree of suspicion, there are some that set off immediate alarm bells. These are so-called dysplastic nevi—atypical moles that have a much higher-than-average potential to become cancerous. People who have dysplastic nevi are at much greater-than-average risk of developing melanoma on other, mole-free parts of their skin.

Most doctors who follow patients with dysplastic nevi regularly and frequently will suggest that the moles be surgically excised so that the tissues can be examined for malignant cells. A dermatologist should remove a mole with a laser only after conclusively determining that it is not cancerous.

The following are considered signs that a mole may be dangerous:

- The mole measures more than about five-eighths of an inch in diameter.

- The mole has recently appeared on a patient over the age of 40. (Most acquired moles show up before middle age.)

- The mole changes in size, shape or color, particularly if it develops irregular borders. (Moles that darken or enlarge with puberty or pregnancy tend to retain their smooth borders.)

- The mole appears to have some whitish, bluish or pinkish areas in it.

- The mole bleeds easily or appears ulcerated.

- Small satellite moles or other lesions appear around an existing mole.

SKIN CARE AFTER LASER REMOVAL OF PIGMENTED LESIONS

Laser removal of pigmented lesions usually involves multiple treatments, separated by six to eight week intervals. Immediately after each treatment, the skin will feel sore, although usually for no more than an hour or two. For one to two weeks, it will appear unsightly, covered with red spots and small contusions that crust over. As the bruises fade, there should be perceptible lightening of the brown spot.

1. Keep the treated areas coated with an antibiotic ointment such as bacitracin or polysporin ointment (not Neosporin, which can cause allergic reactions in some people). Gently clean with soap and water once or twice a day until all the crusting is gone—usually within 10 to 14 days. If you wish, you may cover the areas with a non-stick bandage (Telfa pad).

2. Take acetaminophen (such as Tylenol) to relieve any discomfort or pain. If pain persists past 24 hours, notify your doctor. If there is swelling, apply gel ice packs—or bags of frozen corn or peas—wrapped in a soft cloth to the treated area for 10-15 minutes every hour.

3. You may shower or bathe, but do not rub lased areas with a washcloth. Pat the skin gently dry with a soft towel.

4. You can apply makeup to the treated areas as soon as the crusts have cleared. Be very careful when removing your makeup; rubbing hard will interfere with healing and can lead to permanent changes in your skin's texture.

5. If you are going outside, be sure to apply a broad spectrum sunscreen with SPF 15 or greater to the treated areas. As long as the skin is red or bruised, sun exposure can potentially cause permanent undesirable changes in color.

TINA ALSTER, M.D. & LYDIA PRESTON

6. Treated areas may start to turn more brown (hyperpigment) as they heal. If this happens, inform the doctor who can prescribe bleaching medication to arrest the browning.

CHAPTER SIX

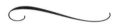

BLASTING OFF TATTOOS

*T*he practice of decorating the body with tattoos dates back to the Stone Age. Archaeologists believe that as long ago as 12,000 BC, cave dwellers slashed their skin during bereavement ceremonies and rubbed ashes into the cuts to create lasting testaments to their grief. Archaeological evidence found in Europe, China, Japan and North Africa indicate that other primitive peoples around the globe ornamented their skin with designs created from plant and mineral pigments injected with crude needles of wood and bone. Tattooing has persisted through the centuries, in every part of the world, suggesting to social scientists that the urge to use one's own skin as a canvas for expressing individuality, artistic sensibility, group affiliation, sexual identity or rebellion from parental authority is a well nigh universal human inclination.

Nearly as universal has been a subsequent regret at having acquired the tattoo and a strong desire to get rid of it. Six thousand-year-old Egyptian mummies show evidence of resolute efforts to remove the works of skin art. Studies today suggest that more than half of all adults with tattoos wish they didn't have them and dermatologists are regularly consulted by patients who want a tattoo removed. One British physician has reported that one or two of his patients each year express thoughts of suicide stemming from despair over an unwanted tattoo.

Many people find they outgrow their tattoos. Robert, in a burst of rebellious youthful self-expression, got three tattoos in less than two years in his early 20s. "They bugged my parents an awful lot," he recalls of his family's appalled reaction to the bright green, red and orange dragon that snaked across his right shoulder, the eagle's head outlined against an orange sun that adorned his left, and the bluebird the size of a watch face on his wrist.

"Then after a while, I found I wasn't as enamored with them as I once was. By the time I got into my 30s, I began to think, 'Gee, I wish there was some way to get rid of them.'"

But as Robert learned when he began to look into it, getting rid of a tattoo is no easy matter. Whether it is a crude, mono-chromatic badge of gang membership or an ornate, multi-hued personal ornament, any tattoo is part of the very structure of the skin. And until the advent of modern cosmetic lasers, vir-tually the only way to remove a tattoo was to remove the skin that contained it.

HOW A TATTOO BECOMES PART OF THE SKIN

The mechanism behind tattooing is simple. The various inks and other coloring agents that make up the design contain different pigments. These are comprised of microscopic parti-cles of some mineral or organic matter. They are introduced into the skin by a sharp instrument that penetrates the epidermis and places the pigment in the dermis.

This sets off an immediate protective response on the part of the skin. Its natural reaction is to try to eliminate the foreign particles by breaking them down—actually dissolving them—so that they can be flushed out through the lymph system. But tattoo pigments are not soluble and the individual pigment particles—while not visible to the eye—are gigantic relative to the skin's own cellular structure. The skin cannot expel them. So the body's defense system does the next best thing: scavenger cells called macrophages engulf each pigment granule, encapsulating it inside a membrane that insulates it from the live cells of the dermis.

Any tattoo represents millions of these pigment-containing macrophages, thickly spread through the dermis. They become permanently lodged in the tightly woven network of collagen and elastic fibers, lying cheek by jowl with tiny nerves, blood vessels and other tissues. There they stay, inert—and permanent.

Nearly 1,500 years ago, a Greek physician named Aetius invented a way to coax pigment-containing macrophages out of the skin. Called salabrasion, Aetius' method is still sometimes used today. It consists of rubbing the tattooed area very hard—to the point of bleeding—with coarse table salt. The resulting wound is then coated with additional salt packed under a surgical dressing. This invites severe inflammation and delays normal healing, forcing the skin to produce copious amounts of serum that gradually weeps out particles of tattoo pigment.

Salabrasion rarely gets rid of more than a fraction of the pigment in any tattoo—and it always leaves a scar. Nonetheless, no one in all of the ensuing centuries came up with anything much better. All other methods, including dermabrasion, deep chemical peeling, bleaching, burning with acids and surgical incision and grafting, also produce scars.

LASERS ON TATTOOS

The first lasers used on tattoos were as destructive as any of the other treatment met hods. The early continuous wave laser systems used to remove tattoo inks from the skin were somewhat more precise in removing pigmented cells, but heat build-up from the continuous beam badly damaged the tissues of the dermis and caused scarring.

The advent of pulsed lasers capable of heating specific targets while sparing adjacent skin revolutionized tattoo removal. Medically, tattoos are regarded as a deep type of pigmented lesion, like the brown spots described in Chapter 5. Laser surgeons eradicate the ink particles in the same manner as they take out the melanin-containing cells that make up brown lesions. And they use the same instruments to do it—the Q-switched ruby, Nd:YAG and alexandrite lasers and the pigmented lesion dye laser (PLDL). These high-powered lasers with their intensely-focused energy blast tattoo pigment into smithereens, creating much tinier entities that the body can eliminate or hide.

Each laser has unique characteristics in terms of wavelength and pulse duration that make it act differently on different tattoo pigments. Different lasers are used to remove different colored pigments, although tattoos of the same color may not always react in the same way, because tattoo pigments may have different chemical compositions. In general, all of the tattoo lasers are effective in removing black or dark blue tattoo ink. But none of the lasers that are currently available to clinical practitioners can remove all of the inks commonly found in multi-colored professional tattoos. For example, the ruby and alexandrite lasers can remove many green inks, but cannot take out red. The Nd:YAG laser does remove red, but cannot usually take out green. The pigmented lesion pulsed dye laser removes reds, oranges and yellows well, but the relatively shallow depth to which its beam penetrates cannot always reach far enough into the dermis to reach deeply placed pigment.

In practice, it is difficult to predict which will be the best laser to use on any given tattoo. Multicolored tattoos usually require treatment with at least two lasers, and it can take even more to totally eradicate all of the inks in some designs.

Given a sufficient array of lasers to handle different pigments, laser tattoo removal is straightforward and relatively uncomplicated. The major drawback is the need for multiple treatments. No laser system can get rid of all of the ink in any tattoo in one laser session. The number of sessions necessary depends on the kinds and amount of pigment that comprise the tattoo and how many colors it contains. The length of time a tattoo has been in the skin can also influence the length of treatment. Some tattoo pigment naturally degrades over the years, so there is somewhat less pigment to remove in older, more faded tattoos and they typically require fewer treatments.

The tattoos that dermatologists are commonly asked to remove fall into four groups, each with slightly different treatment requirements.

PROFESSIONAL. These are usually the most complex tattoos and are always the hardest to remove, particularly if they cover a large area of skin. Even small professional tattoos are commonly multi-hued designs rendered in bright, deeply saturated colors. Each color represents an enormous amount of pigment. The sheer volume of particles dictates multiple laser treatments. Moreover, because professional tattoo inks are made by different manufacturers and tattoo artists often mix different ingredients to make their own unique colors, their chemical composition is usually a mystery. It is sometimes difficult to know which laser system will be most effective and it is almost impossible to predict how many treatments will be needed. It can take anywhere from six to 20 sessions—or even more. The average is eight to ten.

AMATEUR. These are the simplest tattoos in appearance and are usually the easiest to remove. Typically they are plain designs, often self-applied. Medical tattoos sometimes used to mark radiation ports—through which a cancer patient receives radiation treatment—also fall into this category, as do the identity numbers that are sometimes found on former POWs or on concentration camp survivors. They characteristically consist of a single black or blue-black ink, the colors most readily eradicated by laser. Depending on the size and complexity of the design, fading typically takes two to 10 sessions, averaging four to six.

COSMETIC. These are professionally applied tattoos, commonly consisting of red, black or brown pigments that mimic lip, eye or brow liner. Once chiefly employed as an aid to physically-impaired women who find it difficult to apply conventional makeup, cosmetic tattoos have gained increasing popularity in recent years as a carefree way to enhance facial features.

Unfortunately, many women find that these permanent cosmetics are more than they bargained for. Unless applied with an extremely delicate and subtle touch, they can look harsh and overdone—particularly when fashions change and a given makeup style goes out of date. "I looked like Cleopatra," shuddered 54-year-old Sylvia about the heavy black line of eye-liner tattoo that extended well past the outer corner of her eyes and swept up to her brows in two dramatic arcs.

Because the colors in cosmetic tattoos are designed to mimic natural flesh tones, they tend to be less intense than those found in other professional tattoos. The pigment is often a simple homogenous hue and there are usually fewer pigment particles present in the dermis. These factors can make cosmetic tattoos a breeze to remove; often they can be cleared away in a couple of laser sessions.

But some cosmetic tattoos carry a very serious potential complication in that laser pulses can turn certain inks irreversibly black. Many cosmetic tattoo pigments contain a reddish brown substance found in iron rust and chemically known as ferric oxide (Fe_2O_3). Apparently laser impact causes a chemical reaction that instantly changes rust-colored ferric oxide molecules into ferrous oxide (FeO), which is jet black. Thus a woman having maroon-colored lip liner removed can wind up with a dark black line that resembles a thin black pencil mustache after laser treatment.

Because it is impossible to tell from looking whether a tattoo contains ferric oxide, laser surgeons always approach cosmetic tattoos cautiously, usually starting with a single small test pulse. If the spot instantly turns black, the tattoo contains ferric oxide. At that point the patient has two choices. She can leave the tattoo in place, or she can choose to have the surgeon lase the whole tattoo, turn it all black and then have the black pigment removed with further laser treatments. It can take eight or nine treatments, spaced about a month apart, to get rid of all traces of black—if the laser works at all. On some people it does not and then the only remaining option is to have the tattoo surgically excised.

A prudent course is to give the first test spot a month to heal, and then try lasing it. The way it responds will indicate how well the rest of the tattoo will react to further treatment and how long it may take to clear.

Traumatic. These are the marks left by some accident that forcibly introduces foreign debris into the dermis. Common examples are powder blast marks left by a gunshot, particles of asphalt or dirt that become embedded in a person's skin as the result of a fall from a motorcycle or bicycle, or the black marks that people sometimes get if they accidentally puncture their skin with the point of a pencil. Depending on the size and distribution of the particles, it usually takes around two to six laser treatments to clear a traumatic tattoo. Very large particles of foreign matter or bits that have been imbedded particularly deep by an exceptionally violent trauma sometimes cannot be removed at all.

Preoperative Preparation and Considerations

Before starting laser treatment for tattoo removal, here are some of the issues you should bear in mind and discuss specifically with your doctor:

▶ Try to get some estimate of how many treatments will be needed. No doctor can give you a guarantee on this, but tattoo removal can go on for many months—even years—for an especially colorful professional tattoo and you should be prepared. "The guy who did mine was really good. He put 'em on to stay," ruefully observed Robert, whose dragon, eagle and bluebird were reduced to very pale but still discernible shadows after 19 laser sessions.

▶ Tattoos that have been "overtattooed" with additional pigments to hide an unwanted original design may take a particularly long series of treatments to remove because of the exceptionally high volume of pigment particles.

▶ If you recall having had an allergic reaction when you got the tattoo, inform the doctor. Sometimes, by shattering the pigment, the laser may trigger a similar reaction, although this is rare. If you reacted to any pigment with what is known as a granulomatous response, leaving you with bumpy, scar-like tissue under that particular color, it should not be treated with the laser at all; you could have an even more severe allergic reaction to the laser impact. (This is most common with red pigments and should not prevent you from having other colors lased.)

▶ Other than the rare allergic reaction, complications are minimal. The most common are light scarring or textural changes that are the result of many repeated treatments, or transient hypopigmentation. In the latter case, the skin's natural tone lightens because its own pigment (melanin) is destroyed along with the tattoo pigment. The melanin-producing cells cannot keep up with the pace of a long series of treatments. Usually, once the series of laser treatments is over, melanin production returns to normal, bringing back the natural skin color.

▶ You will have to avoid the sun throughout the course of laser treatments. A tan fills the skin with excess melanin which absorbs laser light, reducing the laser beams' ability to reach the underlying tattoo pigments.

► The very high intensity laser pulses used to break up tattoo pigments cause bruising and often some bleeding. These reactions may be more severe in individuals with a tendency toward bleeding disorders. Inform your doctor if you have ever had problems with wound healing, and avoid taking unnecessary anticoagulant medication (i.e. aspirin) prior to surgery.

► Laser impact can trigger a herpes outbreak. Inform your doctor if you have a history of herpes simplex so you can be started on a preventive medication such as Acyclovir.

TREATMENT

The intense pulses from high-energy tattoo lasers can be very painful, particularly in the case of cosmetic tattoos located around the mouth or eyes. "It's like the worst kind of electric shock and a burn at the same time," is how Sylvia described the sensation of being treated to eradicate the dark lines tattooed around her eyes. The laser also seems to inflict a lot of pain on the extremities, where many tattoos are located. Those areas can be numbed with a topical anesthetic or injected with lidocaine. However, many patients say that the pain of the laser is no worse than they recall from when they were tattooed in the first place, and decline any pain killers.

Depending on the size of the tattoo, a treatment session can last anywhere from 5 minutes to an hour, with the surgeon delivering hundreds of rapid-fire laser pulses to the tattooed skin. Each pulse sends a tiny beam of light into the dermis to explode a minuscule amount of tattoo pigment. The blast dislodges the shattered pigment from its macrophage containers and scatters the granules though the dermis. On the surface, immediately after laser impact, a tiny gray-white circle appears, possibly the result of heat-formed steam around the blasted pigment particles. This is quickly followed by the skin turning red and swollen. Sometimes, especially during early sessions when a lot of tattoo pigment is affected, the inner explosion blows up through the surface of the skin, causing pinpoint bleeding.

The exact fate of the eliminated tattoo pigment is not entirely understood. Some of it apparently comes out externally. Occasionally a small amount of tattoo pigment can be found in the scab that forms over the small wounds. However, most of the work of pigment elimination goes on inside. When the laser energy shatters pigment particles and releases them from their membrane-bound macrophages, the tiniest of the resulting bits are apparently carried away and eliminated by the lymph system. The remaining fragments, too large to be carried off, are less noticeable because the laser's extreme heat evidently changes their molecular structure, making them somewhat translucent, and therefore less apparent through the surface of the skin.

Within about two weeks of treatment, all of the pigment particles remaining in the dermis will have been repackaged inside new macrophages. These repackaged pigment particles, along with those that escaped laser impact, are the targets for the next laser treatment six to eight weeks later.

SKIN CARE AFTER LASER REMOVAL OF TATTOOS

Laser removal of tattoos involves multiple treatments, separated by six to eight week time intervals. After each treatment, the skin over the tattoo will blister, then crust over. When the scab drops off and the redness starts to fade, the entire tattoo will appear lighter.

1. Keep the treated areas coated with an antibiotic ointment such as bacitracin or polysporin ointment (not Neosporin, which can cause allergic reactions in some people). Gently clean with soap and water once or twice a day until all the crusting is gone–usually within 10 to 14 days. If you wish, you may cover the areas with a non-stick bandage, such as a Telfa pad.

2. Take acetaminophen (ie., Tylenol) to relieve any discomfort or pain. If pain persists past 24 hours, notify your doctor. If there is any swelling, apply gel ice packs—or bags of frozen corn or peas—wrapped in a soft cloth to the treated area for 10-15 minutes every hour.

3. You may shower or bathe, but do not rub lased areas with a washcloth. Pat the areas gently dry with a soft towel.

4. If you are going outside, be sure to apply a broad spectrum sunscreen with SPF 15 or greater to the treated areas. As long as the skin is blistered, red or bruised, exposure could cause permanent undesirable changes in color.

5. Treated areas may start to hyperpigment—that is, turn brown–as they heal. If this happens, inform the doctor who can prescribe bleaching medication to arrest the browning.

CHAPTER SEVEN

THE NEW LIGHT
ON RED BIRTHMARKS

*O*ne of Alethea's earliest memories is of crying herself to sleep. In family photographs taken when she was little more than a toddler, she stares into the camera with dark solemn eyes set in an unnaturally white, mask-like face. "I looked like a little geisha," she recalls of her mother's inexpert attempts at applying makeup to camouflage the bright red port-wine stain that ran down both of her cheeks from her eyebrows to her chin.

Jonathan's parents didn't try to hide the ruby-colored stain on the left side of his neck. They wouldn't even acknowledge its existence. One of his earliest memories is of his mother averting her eyes from his birthmark. She never talked about it or tried to explain it to him. He says the first time he ever heard anyone say anything at all about his disfigurement was when he reached school-age. Then, the jibes of other children cruelly reinforced the unspoken message he read into his parents' silence: that he was horribly flawed.

Twelve-year-old Anthony has no memory of this incident, but his father will never forget the day he walked into a room and saw his then four-year-old son staring intently into a mirror, spitting into his little hand then rubbing it hard across his face, trying to scrub the port-wine stain from his cheek and forehead.

Surely almost every individual born with a disfiguring birthmark carries a heavy history of such painful memories. Few people in the 20th century Western world believe that port-wine stains are the Devil's handiwork or subscribe to the ancient theory that they stem from a mother's moral transgressions during pregnancy. And yet children with port-wine birthmarks still grow up feeling as outcast as their counterparts in the Middle Ages who were shunned as pariahs. And they may feel just as helpless to change their condition, for until the advent of dermatologic lasers, there was little that any doctor could do for them.

Port-wine stains are one of the two most common types of red birthmarks. The other is a tumor called a hemangioma. Both are caused by abnormal development of blood vessels in the skin. Physicians still do not understand how and why they occur. They cannot be definitively linked to any known birth-defect-causing chemical or toxin. They are not related to trauma in the womb or accidents at the time of birth. Sometimes they are associated with other developmental malformations. Most of the time they just happen.

PORT-WINE STAINS

Port-wine stains are found on three to five out of every 1,000 children born in North America and are located on the face or neck in up to 90 percent of all cases. They apparently form sometime during early fetal life, when for some reason, a group of rogue blood vessels appears spontaneously. The result is a thin mat of abnormally dilated capillaries, clustered together just beneath the surface of the skin in the upper part of the dermis. The mat shows through the surface as a flat red mark with sharply defined borders.

Port-wine stains are usually evident at birth, although initially they may be so pale in color that they do not seem to be serious. In those cases, they are sometimes confused with a temporary disorder called nevus flammeus, nicknamed "stork bite," "salmon patch" or "angel's kiss." These very light pink marks are commonly found on a newborn's forehead, eyelids or nape of the neck. Doctors do not know the cause. Some think they are remnants of the fetal circulatory system. Unlike port-wine stains, the marks fade completely away, usually by the end of the first year.

Port-wine stains, on the other hand, become progressively darker with time. Typically, they grow proportionately with a child, although they may suddenly expand because of changes in the circulatory system or hormonal fluctuations such as those that occur in puberty. As a person continues to age, the vessels grow steadily in diameter and become more "ectatic." This means that they become increasingly convoluted, twisting and turning on themselves into masses that resemble badly knotted balls of twine.

Over the years, this causes steady darkening and thickening of the birthmark. Port-wine stains are usually bright red by the end of childhood, deep claret by early adulthood, and dark purple by middle age. They become raised and develop nodules. The surface becomes pebbly in texture ("cobblestoned" as it is sometimes called) and increasingly hard to disguise with makeup. In many cases, the overgrowth of blood vessels impinges on structures such as the lips, nose or eyes, distorting the features and even interfering with the way they function.

HEMANGIOMAS

Hemangiomas, or "strawberries" as they are sometimes called, are non-cancerous tumors made up of superfluous blood vessels. Unlike the malformed capillaries in a port-wine stain, the excess blood vessels that make up a hemangioma are essentially normal. There are just too many of them in one spot.

Hemangiomas are the most common tumors found on babies, appearing on about one out of every 10 infants, usually in the first few weeks of life. They do not seem to run in families, but do occur with more frequency among fair-skinned children; by the age of one, an estimated 10 to 12 percent of all Caucasian children have a hemangioma. Girls are more commonly affected than boys, in a ratio of three to one.

The hallmark of a hemangioma is rapid growth. It may first appear as a pinpoint-size red dot, a red patch surrounded by pale halo or an area of blanched skin that quickly becomes infiltrated with a network of tiny blood vessels. Once visible, the tumor grows quickly, usually reaching its full size (anywhere from one to six inches or more in diameter) within a few months.

Hemangiomas fall into three categories, depending on how deeply they reach into the skin. A superficial or capillary hemangioma consists of excess capillaries in the upper part of the dermis. As the capillaries proliferate, they form a mass that pushes up the surface of the skin; it becomes a bright scarlet color that deepens to a ruby hue. Although most capillary hemangiomas remain small, from about one-half of a centimeter to five centimeters in diameter, they can quickly grow to the size of a grapefruit or larger.

A venous hemangioma lies deeper in the structure of the skin, with large vessels proliferating in the lower dermis and often infiltrating the subcutaneous fat below; sometimes the mass of blood vessels even invades underlying muscles. Because the vessels lie so deep in the skin, a venous hemangioma may be only slightly raised and it may appear on the surface as more blue than red in color. Or it may be so deep that it neither raises the surface nor imparts any color to the skin at all. (Venous hemangiomas were once called cavernous hemangiomas, but doctors today regard the term as misleading and rarely use it.)

When a hemangioma involves both superficial and deep layers of the skin (both upper and lower dermis), it is called a mixed hemangioma. These may range in color from pink to dark red depending on how close to the surface the top part of the tumor lies.

Although hemangiomas are usually raised (the Greek suffix oma means swelling), the vessels in even a superficial lesion can infiltrate the skin without lifting it. These flat tumors are often dead ringers for port-wine stains. One way to tell the difference is from the patient's history. A port-wine stain is always present at birth, whereas a hemangioma is only present at birth in some 30 percent of affected children.

The explosive growth that characterizes a hemangioma is almost always followed by a long period during which the tumor progressively shrinks. This is called the involution phase and it usually starts by the time an infant is 10 to 12 months old. The hemangioma will at first seem to stabilize and grow at about the same pace as the child. Then it will gradually soften and start to shrink. The red color may fade, and the skin starts to look mottled and grayish.

Involution is a long slow process, lasting many months. But by the time they are five years old, more than half of all children with hemangiomas are completely free of them. Another 20 per cent see their tumors clear up totally by the age of seven. The remaining 30 per cent will usually see their tumor continue to slowly shrink for another five years or so. If a child is not rid of the lesion by the age of nine years, the hemangioma probably will never go away on its own.

A MAGIC BULLET FOR VASCULAR BIRTHMARKS

Neither the abnormal capillaries in a port-wine stain nor the excess vessels that make up a hemangioma serve any useful purpose. They are not needed to deliver blood to living tissues. They are simply anomalies, and there is no reason not to get rid of them—except for the fact that until recently it was all but impossible to do so without significant side effects.

Numerous means have been tried, including excision and skin grafting, radiation, freezing, dermabrasion, electrocautery, injection with steroids or blood vessel–destroying agents. Virtually all of these methods produced either disfiguring scars or complications ranging from infection and hemorrhage to the serious side effects associated with radiation therapy or high doses of steroids. Moreover, no method ever proved much more effective at actually obliterating vascular blemishes than the old Flemish remedy that instructed mothers to lick their children's birthmarks off.

Before there were lasers, the safest and most effective means of dealing with a vascular birthmark was to cover it with opaque makeup. A more extreme version of the same strategy was to tattoo over the lesion with flesh-colored ink. Other than to remove a birthmark or portion of one that was growing in such a way that it threatened a vital organ, most doctors were reluctant to employ any of the more drastic medical techniques.

From the very beginning, experts recognized that laser technology had the potential to change that situation. In the 1960s pioneering physicians began experimentally using the handful of lasers then available to cauterize and thus shut down the blood vessels that constitute port-wine stains and hemangiomas. This was a crude method that damaged other tissues as well as blood vessels, burning and scarring the skin.

The introduction of the argon laser in the early 1970s allowed doctors to target blood vessels more specifically and for the first time in history offered a feasible means of clearing vascular birthmarks. The argon laser emits an intense blue-green light that is absorbed by red, the color of the hemoglobin in red blood cells. When aimed at a port-wine stain, the laser's beam passes though the skin's surface and the blood vessel walls and is absorbed by the red cells. As the light energy is absorbed, it is transformed into heat which destroys the cells and the surrounding vessel walls. The body gradually clears away the dead tissue just as it clears out the cellular debris that causes a bruise.

Unfortunately, some of the argon laser beam's energy is partially absorbed by the skin pigment melanin as it passes through the skin, reducing the energy that is absorbed by hemoglobin. More significantly, heat inside targeted vessels quickly builds up to very high levels and spreads through the skin by conduction. It is difficult to control this heat build-up and as a consequence, tissues next to the target blood vessels are burned. This permanently damages the skin's collagen structure and the result is almost always some degree of scarring, ranging from relatively mild superficial skin lightening to very obvious raised, or hypertrophic, scars. Children proved particularly prone to scarring with the argon laser, which consequently was not used on patients under 17 years of age.

In a 1984 survey, 87 percent of patients treated with an argon laser indicated that they were bothered by the scars the laser left behind. To this day, many people with port-wine stains have smooth shiny masses of thickened scar tissue in areas once treated with the argon laser. Moreover, even among adults who were regarded as successfully treated with the argon laser, most port-wine stains only lightened to a certain degree, because the laser's wavelength only penetrated the upper dermis, leaving deeper vessels in the birthmark unaffected.

Despite its drawbacks, the argon laser remained the treatment of choice for port-wine stains until the advent of a new laser which became commercially available in the mid-1980s— the flashlamp-pumped pulsed dye laser.

The pulsed dye laser was developed specifically to treat children's port-wine stains. Its light passes through a chamber filled with a liquid dye to emit a yellow light that is more readily absorbed by red blood cells than the blue-green light from the argon laser. It is exquisitely tuned to a precise wavelength (585 nanometers) that penetrates just far enough into the dermis to reach the deeper components of a port-wine stain. And the beam is electronically pulsed, flashing on long enough to deliver the maximum energy needed to instantly incinerate blood cells, then shutting off before surrounding tissues burn. The heat never builds up to the extent that it causes the collagen damage that results in a scar. The end result is unmarked skin with a normal surface in both color and texture.

The 585nm pulsed dye laser proved to be the magic bullet for treating port-wine stains. And although it was designed to eradicate the small blood vessels in children's birthmarks, it is now routinely used with impressive results on the larger, more convoluted blood vessels found in adult port-wine stains.

Increasingly, physicians are also using the same laser on hemangiomas, making it the first truly safe and effective means in history for treating disfiguring vascular birthmarks in patients of all ages.

LASER TREATMENT OF PORT-WINE STAINS

As with many other forms of laser surgery, port-wine stain treatment is simple in concept, but often far from easy on patients. The pulsed dye laser is marvelously precise in seeking out and destroying abnormal blood vessels in a birthmark, but it can treat only a small proportion of the tiny, hair's width vessels at a time. Treatments have to be repeated again and again, making for a tediously long course of therapy spread out over many months or years.

At each session, the birthmark is subjected to a series of laser pulses. Each pulse hits a small section of matted blood vessels, almost immediately producing a dark bluish-black spot on the surface of the skin. These marks, each a little larger than the size of a pencil eraser, are little bruises, called purpura. They are caused by destruction of the blood vessels. The pulses are repeated, adjoining but not overlapping one another until the entire birthmark is covered with a pattern of purplish dots.

The laser beam stings on impact, producing a quick pop that is very much like the snap of a rubber band against the skin. Some people say it feels like the prick of a needle, although they readily concede it is far less painful than getting a shot. It can only be felt for an instant. There is also a brief sensation of heat. The spot feels sore and may itch for half an hour or so afterward.

For most people, the pain of each laser pulse is easily tolerable without anesthetic. However, the accumulated pulses—it takes up to several hundred per session for the average-sized birthmark—can add up to considerable discomfort over the course of a typical 20 to 45 minute session. A topical anesthetic cream, rubbed on the skin 30 to 60 minutes before surgery, is usually all that most adults and older children need to alleviate the discomfort; some people also like to take acetaminophen beforehand. (Very small children, who have no idea what is happening to them, usually have a harder time of it; see sidebar on Young Children and Laser Treatment, pages 134–136.)

Afterwards, there may be minor swelling and redness which usually fades within 48 hours. During that time the skin feels somewhat sunburned. It takes another week to 10 days for the bluish purpura to go away, as the body clears away the debris of destroyed tissue. Then, disappointingly, the treated area looks about as red as it did before. This is caused by inflammation, another stage of the healing process. This redness gradually fades over the next few weeks. Sometimes, people will experience mild temporary skin browning (transient hyperpigmentation) over the treated areas; this usually fades by the time of the next treatment six to eight weeks later.

Most patients see dramatic lightening of their birthmarks several weeks after each of the first few sessions, then proportionately less lightening following subsequent sessions. Infants respond the most quickly and completely. The shallow, small-caliber vessels in an immature port-wine stain can be significantly eradicated within as few as four or five sessions. On the whole, children who begin laser treatment as newborns will see what doctors characterize as 80 to 100 percent clearance in about five to 10 sessions. This means that by the time they reach their second birthday, their birthmarks will have faded to a pale, imperceptible pink or have totally disappeared, with the treated skin exactly matching adjacent skin in color and texture.

Progress tends to be slower for older children. In the three to eight-year-old age group, it may take eight to 12 sessions or more to see 80 percent clearing. Above the age of eight, results become more unpredictable—depending on the size and location of the birthmark, as well as a host of other individual factors. Some older children and teenagers, and even some adults, clear up rapidly, seeing 75-85 percent improvement in as few as six sessions. For others, progress is glacial, taking 20 or more treatments to reach the same stage.

It is extremely difficult to predict how many laser sessions will be needed to significantly clear any given port-wine stain beyond that point. Generally speaking, older port-wine stains respond less well to laser treatment because the blood vessels in older stains are deeper, larger and more convoluted. Also, patients with naturally dark skin are generally somewhat slower to respond to laser therapy because the additional melanin in their skin filters some of the laser light. In patients whose birthmarks have been camouflaged by tattooing, the tattoo pigments will also interfere with the laser beam, as will scars from previous argon laser treatment. (Happily, the pulsed dye laser has a beneficial long-term effect on old argon laser scars, acting to flatten the raised portion and to stimulate the growth of normal collagen. See Chapter 9.)

To compensate for the filtering interference of skin pigment or scar tissue, or to affect larger caliber vessels, a surgeon may increase the power of the laser to a higher energy level. This produces more heat per laser pulse, making the treatment somewhat more painful. As one patient, wincing at the feel of higher energy pulses, wryly noted, "They tell you it's going to feel like a rubber band snapping. They just don't tell you how far back they can pull that rubber band."

Most surgeons will continue to treat a birthmark until it is completely gone or until it does not appear to lighten at all following treatment, indicating that the remaining components of the stain are resistant to the laser. This may be because those vessels lie so deep in the dermis that they are beyond range of the laser beam. Or some of them may be too large in caliber to be destroyed by laser action. In areas that have been subjected to many treatments, vessels that have survived repeated laser hits actually get tougher, developing thickened fibrous walls that the beam can no longer readily penetrate.

TREATING HEMANGIOMAS WITH LASERS

Laser treatment of hemangiomas is more problematic than laser treatment of port-wine stains. Because hemangiomas almost always eventually go away on their own, many pediatricians still routinely counsel parents to leave the tumors alone and let nature take its course—at least until the child is past the age of 10. And indeed, there seems to be no urgent reason to remove a small hemangioma if it is located somewhere, such as on the trunk, where it is neither disfiguring in appearance nor threatening to other bodily structures.

However, many times there are compelling medical reasons to remove a hemangioma. Often—usually at the height of the proliferative phase—a lesion becomes ulcerated, its tightly stretched surface pulling open and bleeding. This is painful, and it may lead to an infection or a permanent scar. Moreover, even a medium-sized hemangioma may so greatly stretch the overlying tissues that it leaves a sagging area of excess skin that will remain long after the tumor itself is gone.

Most seriously, a growing hemangioma can impinge on vital structures. If it encroaches on an eye, it will not only obstruct an infant's vision over the short term, but can also threaten permanent sight, either by interfering with visual development or by exerting distorting pressure on the eyeball. A large hemangioma near the ear can cause temporary hearing loss; hearing impairment that persists past the age of one year will hamper speech development. A hemangioma near the nose can block nasal passages. Near the throat, it may obstruct the airway—a potentially life-threatening complication.

Aside from purely medical considerations, the overriding motive to have a hemangioma removed is concern that the disfiguring growth will lead to emotional problems, particularly once a child reaches school age and is subjected to the scrutiny of peers. Even very young children can become extremely self conscious about these tumors. One doctor has reported the distressing account of a four-year-old girl so determined to get rid of a hemangioma that she took matters into her own hands and tried to cut it off with a pair of nail scissors.

Laser treatment of hemangiomas is virtually identical to that for port-wine stains. The same 585nm pulsed dye laser is used in a series of sessions, with each treatment eliminating a proportion of the proliferating vessels that make up the tumor. Treatments are repeated at monthly intervals. In most cases, the goal is not to eradicate the tumor, but to keep it within a manageable, less invasive size until it starts to go away on its own.

Superficial (capillary) hemangiomas respond the best. If laser treatment is started at the first sign of the tumor developing—when it is still thin and flat—there is a good chance that the laser can remove enough of the excess vessels to prevent the tumor from ulcerating and bleeding, and restrain its growth so that it will not impinge on other parts of the body.

Deep (venous) and mixed hemangiomas are more difficult to treat, because the vessels deep in the dermis are beyond the laser's range. In these cases, it is still beneficial to remove the more superficial component of the tumors with the laser and attempt to minimize the deeper portions with anti-inflammatory steroids—either taken by mouth or injected directly into the tumor. This combination treatment has the advantage of reducing at least part of the tumor's bulk with the laser, while reducing the amount of side effect-causing steroids that would otherwise be used.

The Psychological Impact

To whatever extent a port-wine stain or hemangioma clears up following laser treatment, the changes that patients experience go far beyond the superficial appearance of their skin. Overwhelmingly, anyone with a disfiguring birthmark will say that it has been the central, dominating fact of his or her life. Inevitably, there are profound psychological ramifications as the mark fades.

Sometimes the consequences are immediate and dramatically positive—as is very often the case with children. Painfully shy and withdrawn youngsters blossom into outgoing, self-confident personalities. Teenagers who have been too timid to make friends develop spirited social lives. Grades at school skyrocket. "I feel his true character is showing now, not just what people see on his face," said Anthony's father, of the changes he observed as his son's birthmark lightened.

With remarkable consistency, patients describe a sense of being able to "get on" with their lives or getting their lives "back" after getting rid of a birthmark. A large hemangioma, which for some reason never spontaneously involuted, had engulfed 33-year-old Craig's left ear since childhood. As a series of laser treatments gradually reduced the size of the tumor and restored his ear to a more normal appearance, Craig was jubilant. "I'm living a whole new life," he crowed.

For other patients, the loss of a birthmark triggers conflicting feelings, including grief, fear, anger, sadness and guilt. People expect these strong emotions in response to devastating life changes such as bereavement or divorce. But such feelings can be deeply bewildering to those who finally secure the one thing they have yearned for all of their lives. "The emotional floodgates have burst open," said Jonathan, who like a number of other birthmark patients sought psychiatric counseling to help him cope with the changes he experienced. "Suddenly I have to deal with how much of my personality is tied up with feeling deformed."

"Such feelings are not so strange when you think about them," said Alethea, "for the loss of a birthmark is, in part, a loss of identity, of one's very self." Crying softly as she recounted the deep pain that other people's reactions to her port-wine stain had once caused her, she said she felt hurt anew by their enthusiastic acceptance of her new face after three years of laser treatment. "I'm offended because it implies that I was unacceptable before."

It's complicated, agreed Anthony. Unusually open and active for a child with a disfiguring birthmark, Anthony admitted shedding copious private tears over the years. Yet he always did well academically, made friends readily, and managed to come up with bluntly effective juvenile strategies for countering the stares and taunts of other kids.

"He fakes them out," hooted his younger brother. "He tells them he got it in a nuclear accident and flies DIE if they land on his cheek."

"It's good when I play football," laughed Anthony. "Guys on other teams sometimes don't want to touch me, so a lot of times

I don't get tackled."

Anthony was apprehensive about laser surgery. "I was scared people wouldn't like me any more if I changed and became different." So he polled neighbors and friends to find out what everybody else thought. Aside from his brother and a few young peers, who pronounced his port-wine stain "cool" because it made him look like the comic book villain "Two-Face," the response was "Go for it." Which, despite his fears, was what he knew he wanted for himself.

A year later, after five laser treatments had turned his birthmark light pink, Anthony still had mixed feelings. "I'm glad I'm doing it. I'm glad it's working. But I wish I had it done when I was a baby and it was all over now," he confided wearily. "I just wish this had never happened to me period."

Probably no aspect of laser surgery is as emotionally charged as the question of how to help very young children, who cannot understand why they are being subjected to it, cope with the trauma associated with laser treatment. There is no doubt from a medical point of view that the earlier a birthmark is treated, the better. When started in early infancy, laser surgery can eradicate even a large port-wine stain without a trace by the time the child reaches his or her second birthday. The procedure is totally safe.

The only question is how much, if any, anesthetic should be used. The 585nm flashlamp-pumped pulse dye laser used for treating birthmarks is considered to be the least painful of any skin laser. The sensation of an individual pulse is only a fraction of what a child feels from an immunization. Because the discomfort is so minor, adults are routinely treated without any pain-killing medication other than topical numbing creams. Many don't even bother with those.

But laser therapy is much more traumatic for children. Although the laser is not excruciating—particularly if the skin has been pre-treated with a numbing agent—its repeated laser pulses still hurt. And the procedure is very frightening to youngsters. The powerful laser beam poses a danger to eyesight, so the child's eyes must be covered, which can be extremely scary. And children have to be held very still, which is also upsetting.

It is upsetting for their mothers and fathers as well. Seeing a weeping, struggling child being held down to undergo laser treatment is wrenching. Many parents have understandable concerns about the long-term psychological effects on their children.

Nonetheless, laser surgeons and pediatricians are extremely cautious about anesthetizing or sedating children to help them through the procedure. The reason is that infants and young children are much more likely than adults to suffer serious complications from any form of anesthesia or sedation. The risks are magnified by the fact that laser treatments must be repeated every couple of months; experts worry that repeatedly anesthetizing a young child could adversely affect neurological development. They argue that using anesthesia to alleviate the minor and transient pain the child experiences is not worth the medical risk.

This is a subject that parents of children with birthmarks must discuss thoroughly with their physicians. Together, parents and doctors can weigh the immediate stress of laser treatment against the emotional pain that older children experience when they become aware of their disfigurement and of other peoples' reactions to it. Parents are often reassured to learn that in laser centers where many children are treated, most babies and toddlers bounce back instantly from laser sessions and do not exhibit any signs of distress afterwards.

School-age children, from about the age of eight years up, use topical numbing creams and generally claim that laser surgery is not that bad. According to 12-year-old Anthony, "It feels more, like, weird. Afterwards, it feels like a sunburn and I have to put on an ice pack." A young girl, undergoing treatment for a birthmark on the left side of her mouth, added, "You get used to it and then it doesn't hurt much."

On the whole, it is children from about two to seven or eight years old who seem to be the most distressed by laser treatment. They are too young to fully understand what is being done, yet they are old enough to remember previous treatments and anticipate future ones. As a result, they sometimes become so panicky that their fears actually magnify the pain of surgery. Parents of children in that age group should carefully review their options with a qualified pediatric anesthesiologist. Along with the limited use of sedatives, there are a number of pain-reducing medications and anxiety-relieving techniques that can help a child better tolerate the procedure without resorting to heavy anesthesia. Sometimes parents decide to wait and initiate laser treatments when the child is older and more personally motivated to get rid of the birthmark.

SKIN CARE AFTER LASER TREATMENT FOR PORT-WINE STAINS AND HEMANGIOMAS

The lased areas of the skin are very fragile while the blue-grey purpura (bruises) are present and must be treated with extreme care.

1. Apply bacitracin or polysporin ointment (not Neosporin, which causes allergic reactions in some people) to the treated area and cover it with a nonstick bandage (Telfa pad with adhesive) one to two times a day until the purpura have faded (seven to ten days).

2. To relieve any swelling, apply a gel ice pack—or a bag of frozen peas or corn—wrapped in a soft cloth to affected areas, every hour for 10 to 15 minutes at a time.

3. Take acetaminophen (ie., Tylenol) to relieve any discomfort or pain; if pain persists past 24 hours, notify your doctor.

4. Do not take aspirin or any aspirin-containing medicines, or drink alcohol during the healing period (one to two weeks or until the bruising has completely disappeared).

5. You may shower or bathe, but do not rub lased areas with a washcloth. Pat gently dry with a towel. The skin is extremely delicate over the bruised areas and it can easily be broken with vigorous rubbing.

6. Protect treated areas from sun exposure, which can lead to permanent skin changes. Use a broad spectrum sunscreen with SPF 15 or higher throughout your course of treatment.

7. Avoid contact sports and do not go swimming as long as purpura are present.

8. You may wear makeup as soon as the purpura and swelling subside. Use extreme care in removing it; rubbing too hard can injure the skin and may lead to changes in its texture.

CHAPTER EIGHT

GETTING THE RED OUT:
ROSACEA, SPIDER VEINS, CHERRY SPOTS,
AND OTHER BLEMISHES

*I*t starts innocuously—a brief reddening of the face, a warm flush that suffuses the cheeks, nose, chin or forehead. Almost as soon as it appears, it fades away. Only to reappear after a hot meal or a cold beer, a jog on a summer's day, or a winter's morning on the ski slopes. Your face turns bright red. It gets hot. It feels uncomfortable. And it's embarrassing. Others may comment on your scarlet cheeks or wonder privately if you've had too much to drink.

Even so, your red face may not seem all that significant. After all, most people occasionally blush in embarrassment or turn pink with exertion. But persistent, deep, hair-trigger flushing is often the first symptom of rosacea, a chronic skin disorder that affects an estimated 13 million Americans. Rosacea, or "red nose," as some people call it, is not a grave disease. But the popular association of a red face with ill health or heavy drinking makes it stigmatizing. And the condition can worsen to a degree that it actually becomes disfiguring—

producing hard, raised bumps on the cheeks or a huge, bulbous claret-colored nose.

"I used to get beet red, and people were always asking me if I was OK or if any thing was wrong. Once at my office, someone told me to sit down and he would go get the company nurse. He thought I was having a stroke!" recalled Maryanne, 47. "And then the bumps. I thought, what's this? Acne? At my age?"

Rosacea is one of the most common of a number of skin reddening conditions that doctors classify as acquired vascular lesions—"acquired" because they are not present at birth. Yet they are similar to vascular birthmarks such as port-wine stains in that they get their color from abnormal blood vessels lying directly beneath the surface of the skin. And they can be removed with the same laser that is used on red birthmarks— the 585nm flashlamp-pumped pulsed dye laser that works by selectively destroying the aberrant vessels, leaving the surface unscathed.

Acquired vascular lesions sometimes appear as a sign of an underlying medical condition or in response to an injury. More commonly they are merely benign superficial anomalies. Just about everybody eventually gets a few as they age, acquiring "spider veins" on the face or legs, bright red "cherry spots" on the trunk, or patchy, chronically ruddy skin on the neck or chest.

Whether caused by disease, injury or the wear and tear of time, there are many ways superficial blood vessels can show up as blemishes on the surface. Most commonly they manifest themselves in one of three ways: as flat red lines or blotches, as raised red bumps or as red or blue leg veins.

Red lines or blotches on the skin come from permanently dilated superficial blood vessels. The medical term for them is telangiectasias. Patients usually refer to them as "spider veins" or "broken veins." They can show up anywhere on the body in a multitude of patterns, from isolated filaments to dense nets encompassing broad areas of skin. Often they occur in response to hormonal changes, such as those associated with pregnancy, menopause or the use of birth control pills. They sometimes appear at the site of an infection or an injury, or as a side effect to an illness. Sun damage, which degrades the skin's fibrous collagen support structure, allowing little vessels to expand easily, is a major contributing factor.

Telangiectasias are small visible vessels, ranging in diameter from .1 millimeter (mm)—roughly a hair's width—to about 1 mm (not much thicker than fishing line or darning thread) or even larger. Much smaller vessels, too tiny to be seen with the naked eye, may also become permanently dilated, producing a diffuse background blush (called erythema) in which there are no visible lines. Very often people who acquire telangiectasias also have erythema in the same area. The visual effect is pink to red skin, superimposed with tiny red lines.

Physicians can remove telangiectasias with sclerotherapy or electrodessication. In sclerotherapy, the blood vessel is injected with a foreign substance such as a concentrated saline (or salt) solution that wounds the vessel, causing it to scar internally and close off. Blood can no longer get in, so the discoloration disappears. Sclerotherapy is the routine treatment for visible leg veins and is also used at other body sites on large caliber telangiectasias greater than 1 mm in diameter—about the same as a sewing needle.

Electrodessication is performed with a very fine, electrically heated needle that is inserted into the vessel every two to three millimeters, evaporating each little section. Most commonly employed on small vessels, electrodessication requires great skill and experience on the part of the physician. But even in very skilled hands, it is unpredictable and often results in tiny white puncture scars where the needle has penetrated the skin.

Small caliber telangiectasias (up to 1 mm in diameter) respond extremely well to treatment with the 585nm pulsed dye laser. Laser surgery is also the only effective way to remove the microscopic vessels that produce erythema. The red skin is subjected to a series of laser pulses that penetrate the epidermis and blood vessel walls to incinerate the red blood cells and thus destroy the vessels from the inside out. As in other forms of treatment with this laser, each pulse stings on impact, much like the snap of a rubber band. Most people do not need anesthetic; those who do usually find that a topical numbing cream rubbed on the skin 30 to 60 minutes before surgery is sufficient.

Destruction of the vessels immediately produces dark bluish-black bruises (purpura) on the skin surface. The treated skin will be covered with a pattern of closely spaced dots about the size of a pencil eraser or slightly larger. The dots may touch, but they should not overlap; areas of skin treated with overlapping laser pulses may heal poorly with changes in texture, or even scarring. The spots remain sore and may itch for half an hour or so afterwards. There is also minor swelling and redness which feels like a sunburn; it usually subsides within 48 hours.

It takes a week to 10 days for the bluish purpura to fade as the body clears away the shattered blood vessels and other cellular debris. Some patients experience temporary skin browning (transient hyperpigmentation) over the treated areas; this usually fades within six to eight weeks.

The most common forms of telangiectasia that doctors now treat with laser surgery are:

ESSENTIAL TELANGIECTASIAS. These are simple thread-like lines that may occur anywhere on the body. In some cases the lines branch out like trees; these are called arborizing telangiectasias. When not related to some underlying disorder, essential telangiectasias are usually the result of progressive sun-damage. They are very common on the face, especially around the nose and on the cheeks and chin. Grouped together in fish-net configurations, they impart a deep florid look to the skin.

It usually takes only one treatment with the pulsed dye laser to eliminate the telangiectasias in a given area. However, in sections of skin where there is dense matting of vessels, the pattern of laser pulses may leave a latticework of unaffected vessels behind; those are treated in a second session six to eight weeks later. Large-caliber telangiectasias may also require a second or even third treatment. In those cases, the first laser treatment may have injured the vessel enough to shrink it but not destroy it entirely; additional treatment should finish the job. Large telangiectasias (those more than about 1 mm in diameter) are minimally affected by laser treatment and are best treated with sclerotherapy.

ROSACEA. Rosacea is a chronic facial skin disorder, most commonly affecting fair-skinned individuals, particularly women. It is a condition of middle age, typically appearing in a person's 30s or 40s. Rosacea is progressive, with symptoms accumulating over the course of several years. It first manifests itself as unusually persistent flushing in response to stress or exertion. The flushing worsens as blood vessels in the "blush areas" of the cheeks, nose and chin, become weakened and permanently stretched. Even people who have been religious about sun protection notice that their faces seem to be taking on a kind of rough, weather-beaten appearance.

Over time, the flushing becomes even more pronounced, with these uncomfortable episodes lasting longer each time. The skin always looks red and irritated; it becomes interlaced with networks of visible veins. Little hard red bumps (papules) or pus-filled pimples appear over the red areas. It is because of these bumps that rosacea is sometimes called "acne rosacea" or "adult acne." In extreme cases, most commonly in men, the bumps on the nose enlarge into distorting nodular growths—the condition called rhinophyma (see Chapter 4).

No one knows precisely what causes rosacea, and it cannot be cured. However, it can be controlled and its progress arrested though medication and lifestyle changes. Usually a combination of topical and oral antibacterial medicines are used to treat the pimple-like bumps. (Conventional acne medicines such as Retin-A do not work and may actually make the condition worse.) Doctors also advise patients to avoid anything that might trigger flushing. These aggravating factors are different for different people, but they include hot food or drinks, alcohol, spicy condiments, stress, sunlight and extremes in temperature. People who turn bright red when they exercise can control flushing by sucking on ice chips or drinking icy cold water.

The 585nm pulsed dye laser has proved to be enormously successful in clearing the chronically dilated small blood vessels of rosacea. It usually takes two to three treatments, at six to eight week intervals. As well as eliminating the unattractive vessels, the laser also appears to have a beneficial impact on the course of the disorder itself—although doctors don't fully understand the reasons behind this any more than they do the biological processes that cause rosacea in the first place. Nonetheless, a number of physicians have observed that after treatment with a pulsed dye laser, rosacea patients seem to have far fewer papules and pustules—or none at all—and do not need antibiotics to maintain their clear skin. Laser treatment also apparently stimulates the growth of new collagen fibers in the dermis; the resulting stronger, more normal collagen network seems to retard the formation of additional abnormal vessels.

POIKILODERMA. This is a sun-induced disorder in which the skin thins and becomes permanently discolored—a patchy red from telangiectasias, with overlying areas of brownish hyperpigmentation. The skin is very fragile and develops very fine, tissue-paper like wrinkles. Poikiloderma usually affects the delicate, vulnerable skin on the sides of the neck and upper chest. In those areas it is called poikiloderma of Civatte and it is very common among women with a history of excessive sun exposure, particularly women who have been exposed to sunlight after spraying their neck and chest with perfumes or colognes.

The telangiectasias of poikiloderma of Civatte can be eradicated with the 585nm pulsed dye laser, but it is a long, grueling and costly process. Because the affected areas are usually so extensive, it takes from four to six (or even more) lengthy treatment sessions, spaced six to eight weeks apart to get out all the red. Recovery is extremely slow and during the entire course of treatment, the skin will probably look worse than ever— weirdly mottled with variations in color reflecting different stages of healing. Also, because the affected skin is so frail, it is at very high risk for scarring and textural changes. It is essential that anyone contemplating laser treatment for poikiloderma seek out the most experienced physician available. (Insist on seeing before and after treatment pictures of patients that the doctor has treated for the same condition.)

If laser surgery does not prove to be a feasible option, the best treatment for poikiloderma is to avoid additional damage by scrupulously protecting all affected areas from the sun. Consistent use of bleaching creams containing hydroquinone or other bleaching agents may fade brown, hyperpigmented areas; sometimes ointments containing anti-inflammatory corticosteroids can reduce the redness.

CHERRY SPOTS AND OTHER RAISED RED DOTS

There are several common acquired vascular lesions consisting of closely packed collections of dilated blood vessels that push up the epidermis to create a red or purplish bump. They can be removed through electrosurgery, but the procedure destroys the overlying epidermis as well as the vascular component of the lesion, usually leaving a small scar. Successful treatment with the 585nm flashlamp-pumped pulsed dye laser destroys only the abnormal vessels; the skin heals with the same color and texture as the skin surrounding it.

CHERRY ANGIOMAS. Also called cherry spots, ruby spots or senile angiomas, these are the most common of all acquired vascular anomalies, occurring in every ethnic group and with equal frequency among men and women. Cherry spots are usually a sign of advancing age. Most people start showing a few cherry angiomas in their 30s, and continue to acquire additional ones through the years. They are also sometimes brought on by hormonal changes; about five percent of all pregnant women acquire them, usually in the first trimester.

Cherry angiomas usually occur on the trunk, arms, legs and neck; rarely on the face, hands or feet. They form in the little capillaries of the dermal papillae—the tiny projections that constitute the top portion of the dermis (the papillary dermis). As people get older, some of the capillaries in the papillae develop bulbous swellings and torturous knots that appear on the surface as bright red to deep burgundy-colored, round or oval papules.

Laser treatment of cherry angiomas usually consists of subjecting each lesion to a single laser pulse. This turns the spot blackish and surrounds it with a tender, slightly swollen, reddish purple bruise (purpura). As the bruise fades, the raised portion of the angioma flattens out and gradually loses color. Within a few weeks, small spots usually disappear as if they had never existed. Larger lesions typically shrink, but do not disappear entirely because only a portion of the abnormal vessels can be removed at once. It usually takes another one to two additional laser treatments, spaced six to eight weeks apart, to eradicate them.

SPIDER ANGIOMAS. "Spiders" are composed of a central arteriole (a tiny artery) connected to a network of tiny vessels (telangiectasias) that radiate out like the legs of a spider. The center is raised; if you press on it, the legs branch out. Spiders most typically appear in young children, peaking between the ages of seven and 10, but as many as 15 percent of all adults have them as well. They occur frequently in pregnant women, usually appearing in the first trimester.

Pregnancy-related spiders typically disappear within six weeks after delivery. Others are more persistent or essentially permanent. It usually takes one or two sessions with the pulsed dye laser to get rid of a spider angioma; the laser pulse destroys the tiny central vessel, depriving the "legs" of blood and eliminating them as well.

PYOGENIC GRANULOMA. This is an acquired vascular tumor that very closely resembles a small hemangioma (see Chapter 7). It is caused by a proliferation of tiny dermal vessels, creating a painless, rapidly growing red or purple nodule ranging from a few millimeters to several centimeters in diameter. It is a very common disorder, most frequently seen in children and young adults, very often on the lip or nose. Pyogenic granulomas also may occur at the site of any trauma or infection; they have been known to appear following dermabrasion, Retin-A treatment, hair transplantation and laser resurfacing surgery. They frequently crop up within adult port-wine stains.

Pyogenic granulomas are very fragile. They easily break open and bleed—so frequently that the condition has been called the "band-aid disease" because so many patients wind up with band-aids stuck on their faces. In part because the vessels that cause them may extend very deeply into the skin and continue to grow, these lesions respond very unpredictably to laser treatment. Sometimes they clear up very well; other times they remain essentially unaffected. Sometimes doctors recommend surgically excising the raised portion of the lesion, then lasing the remaining deep vessels.

VENOUS LAKE. Most commonly found on older men, venous lakes are small purple or bluish papules that typically appear on the lips or ears. They are caused by a knot of tiny, thin-walled, bulging veins located deep in the skin (in the lower or middle dermis). They are soft to the touch; if you press one with your finger, it will empty of blood and momentarily disappear. They may bleed if traumatized.

Smaller venous lakes—up to about a quarter of an inch in diameter—respond best to laser treatment. They can usually be removed with one to three treatments. Larger lesions are more difficult to eliminate; it may take many more laser sessions and deeper portions may remain behind.

LEG VEINS

Among the most detested of common skin blemishes, unsightly red, blue or purple leg veins, are also among the most difficult lesions to remove by any means. Typically larger in caliber than telangiectasias located elsewhere on the body, visible leg veins also tend to have thicker walls and a somewhat more complex structure than other superficial vessels. They are usually fed by much larger, faulty vessels lying deep beneath the skin. Sometimes these feeder vessels are small arteries; they produce wiry looking red telangiectasias. More commonly, the defective fountainhead vessels are varicose veins—abnormally widened veins with damaged valves that cannot perform their intended function, which is to help blood that has flowed down into the lower extremities circulate back up to the heart. There are numerous possible reasons for valves to give way, including inborn weakness, disease, hormonal changes and the stresses imposed by weight gain, pregnancy or long periods of standing. Blood collects in the affected vein and swells it.

A varicose vein may be visible on the surface as a thick rope, popped up well above the surface, or it may be buried so deeply beneath the skin that it cannot be detected at all. Wherever it lies, a varicose vein connected to smaller, superficial veins in the dermis is likely to turn those vessels into cord-like blue or purple telangiectasias. Doctors theorize that the pressure of blood emanating from the deeper vessels forces the superficial ones open and keeps them permanently dilated. The pressure may also cause various organic changes that generate additional vessels—sometimes extensive networks of them.

Because none of the lasers in common use for other vascular lesions has so far proved to have much of an effect on leg veins, most practicing physicians favor the tried-and-true approach to treating them—sclerotherapy. There are several potential side effects. About 30 percent of patients will experience temporary skin browning (hyperpigmentation) of the treated areas. This is caused by leakage of red blood cells from the damaged vessels and usually clears up within six months if the skin is not exposed to the sun or subjected to injury. Another possible side effect is so-called telangiectatic matting in which a small network of telangiectasias appear around the site of the injection. Sometimes those small vessels respond well to treatment with the 585nm pulsed dye or other vascular-specific laser.

A number of doctors and researchers have tried to develop alternate new devices specifically designed to treat leg veins. Modified versions of the 585nm pulsed dye laser employing different wavelengths and pulse durations have shown some promise in experimental trials. So too has a patented laser-like apparatus called the Photoderm, which while employing a different form of light, works in a similar fashion to the lasers that are used to treat vascular malformations. So far, neither of those instruments or other therapies have conclusively demonstrated their superiority to sclerotherapy in most situations.

In any event, no matter how effective any treatment may be, leg veins almost inevitably recur in susceptible individuals, because without surgery to tie off the feeding vessels, doctors cannot stem the high pressure flow that leads to formation of the smaller visible vessels. Eventually, treated veins either re-open or successor veins pop up in their place. Usually it takes regular treatment to keep them reduced to a cosmetically acceptable level. "I figure it's maintenance," shrugged one woman. "Like cutting your hair."

WHAT ON EARTH ARE THOSE SPOTS?

The immediate aftermath of a session with the 585nm flash-lamp-pumped pulsed dye laser is not pretty, especially if it has been aimed at your face. "God, I looked like an alien," groaned Maryanne, describing the pattern of dark purple dots that spread over her cheeks and nose like a pointillist butterfly. "It's bizarre looking," agreed Ellen who, like Maryanne, was treated for rosacea. "I scared the mailman. He had a package he wanted me to sign for, but he was afraid to hand me his pen."

For most patients, the very distinct and obvious bruises the 585nm pulsed dye laser leave behind constitute the most significant drawback to its use. The laser was designed expressly to destroy very fine superficial blood vessels from the inside out, and the greyish-blue or purple purpura that show up as a result are a sign that it has indeed done its job. The color comes from cellular debris comprised of shattered vessels and blood cells that have spilled into the enveloping dermis. The body's own scavenging mechanism gradually cleans up this organic litter, leaving the skin undamaged and unmarked. Scarring or other permanent skin changes are almost unheard of—provided the physician has not mistakenly laid successive laser pulses on top of one another or used an inappropriate laser energy. But it can take 10 days or more for the unattractive dark spots to fade, and brownish or yellowish marks may linger for months afterward. Understandably, patients want to know if there isn't another way to get rid of their unsightly red facial veins.

In fact there is an alternative: treatment with any one of a number of continuous wave (CW) or so-called quasi-pulsed lasers that act in a slightly different way to eliminate superficial blood vessels. There are a number of these lasers; the most familiar ones are the argon, the argon-pumped tunable dye, the KTP, the copper bromide, the krypton and the copper vapor lasers. They are refined versions of the older continuous-wave instruments first used in dermatology. Those lasers frequently left terrible burn scars due to uncontrolled heat build-up in the tissues. The successor machines are equipped with special shuttering or scanning devices, often coupled with precision fiberoptic aiming technology, that give physicians much greater control over the laser beam. A number of dermatologists employ continuous wave lasers on facial veins—particularly on large caliber vessels that may not respond as well to the 585nm pulsed dye laser.

A doctor traces the target vessel with the CW laser beam, which coagulates the blood, closing off the vessel and shutting it down without creating a bruise. If the procedure is performed correctly, it should leave no sign at all on the surface—other than the desired blanching of the red line. But, inside, a very small thread of fibrous scar tissue will permanently replace the vanished capillary, although it should not be perceptible to the eye or detectable to the touch. The drawback to all continuous wave laser therapy is that this fibrotic tissue sometimes is detectable, particularly if the operating physician is not highly skilled. The question for any patient is whether the immediate convenience of continuous wave laser therapy justifies the small, but nonetheless real, risk of even minor permanent changes in the skin's appearance or texture.

SKIN CARE AFTER LASER TREATMENT FOR RED BLEMISHES

The lased areas will be covered with blue-grey purpura (bruises). The skin over those spots is very fragile and must be treated with extreme care.

1. Apply bacitracin or polysporin ointment (not Neosporin, which causes allergic reactions in some people) to the treated area and cover with a nonstick bandage (Telfa pad with adhesive) once or twice a day until the purple purpura have faded (seven to 10 days.)

2. Take acetaminophen (Tylenol) to relieve any discomfort or pain; if pain persists past 24 hours, notify your doctor.

3. Do not take aspirin or any aspirin-containing medicines, or drink alcohol during the healing period (one to two weeks, or until the bruising has completely disappeared).

4. You may shower or bathe, but do not rub lased areas with a washcloth. Pat gently dry with a towel. The skin is extremely delicate over the bruised area and it can easily be broken with vigorous rubbing.

5. To relieve any swelling, apply a gel ice pack—or a bag of frozen peas or corn—wrapped in a soft cloth, every hour for 10 to 15 minutes at a time.

6. Protect treated areas from sun exposure which can lead to permanent skin changes. Use a broad spectrum sunscreen with SPF 15 or higher throughout your course of treatment.

7. Avoid contact sports and do not go swimming while purpura are present.

8. You may wear makeup after a few days. Use extreme care in removing makeup; rubbing too hard can injure the skin and lead to permanent changes in its texture.

CHAPTER NINE

SCARS, BURNS AND STRETCH MARKS

O n that early spring morning, Elizabeth's life changed forever in a flash. The 31-year-old corporate executive was getting ready for work. She had just stepped out of the shower, combed some conditioner through her damp hair and wrapped her head in a towel. She slipped on a short terry cloth robe and went into the kitchen to put on some water for tea.

She has no memory of what happened next. Perhaps her balky gas stove sent out a spark or a lick of flame; there is some evidence that a burner malfunctioned, so there may have been a small explosion. Whatever the cause, it instantly set ablaze Elizabeth's robe and the towel on her head.

"I think there were some fumes or chemicals in the hair conditioner that caught fire," she speculated a year and a half later, still trying to understand how she could have turned so quickly into a living torch. "I was a fireball," she said.

Rescued by neighbors who heard her screams, and helicoptered unconscious to the hospital, Elizabeth spent the next six weeks in a coma as doctors fought to save her life, and her grievously injured body struggled to repair itself. Third degree burns, in which all layers of the skin are consumed down to the muscle, covered her body from her scalp to her fingers, torso and thighs. Burns that deep and extensive are among the worst calamities that can befall the human organism. The consequences include shock, circulatory and respiratory collapse, kidney and heart failure and massive infections. A decade ago, Elizabeth would surely have died.

She did not because physicians today are highly adept at saving the lives of patients like her. Armed with potent drugs, sophisticated surgical techniques and expanded medical knowledge, they are well-equipped to thwart the life-threatening complications of serious burns or other grossly destructive wounds. Unfortunately, they have far fewer tools to counter the disfiguring scars that are the life-long aftereffects of such devastating injuries.

As Elizabeth's burns healed, gnarled discolored scars grew over her face and frame. Doctor after doctor carefully explained the limits of their skills in restoring her appearance with skin grafts and plastic surgery. Their prognostications drove her to the verge of suicide. "I was so downhearted, so exhausted and so tired of the whole medical profession. I thought to myself, if any of these guys tells me one more time 'We can't make you the way the way you were,' I'll be in jail for assault. They trot that line out all the time. If you ask any question, the first thing they say is, 'Of course, we can't make you look the way you used to.' It's infuriating. I'm not a fool. I know what they can't do. I want to know what they can do."

Before long, Elizabeth learned that in the darkness of her expectations, there was at least one glimmer of light: the beam of the surgical laser. Doctors are now beginning to recognize that dermatologic lasers can have a tremendous impact on the lives of burn victims and other people with equally terrible scars. In the short history of laser skin surgery, practicing physicians and laboratory researchers alike have discovered—sometimes stumbling on the knowledge by accident—that laser light, properly wielded, has surprising, salutary effects on scar tissue. Lasers cannot literally erase scars, but they can relieve the intense discomfort of persistently painful or itching scars, flatten and fade the color from raised red scars, shrink hard, overgrown keloids, and transform disfiguring fibrous burn scars into tissue more closely approximating the feel and appearance of normal skin.

"It's given me hope," said Elizabeth.

THE MYSTERIOUS PROCESS OF WOUND REPAIR

Laser surgeons cannot explain exactly how their instruments work to alter scars and give badly wounded people hope. Indeed, medical science has only incomplete knowledge of precisely what scars are and how they form, even though the basic mechanics of skin repair following an injury are easy to discern. When skin is wounded, it puts itself back together by producing new cells to replace those that have been destroyed. Cells lying just below and to the sides of the damaged tissue replicate themselves to produce new tissue just like the original. Superficial damage such as minor scrapes, shallow cuts, or mild burns that reach only part way into the dermis heal quickly, usually without leaving a mark.

A scar forms when an injury extends so deeply into the dermis that it destroys or cuts completely through a section of the fibrous collagen and elastin network that make up the flexible scaffolding of the skin. A scab, composed of dried blood, serum and other cellular matter, forms over the raw surface and under its protective shell. The skin goes to work to cover the gap with a new epidermis and bridge it with new collagen.

Working from intact tissue around the wound and within surviving hair follicles, the skin generates epidermal cells that migrate over the laceration to create a new surface. At the same time, it sends out new fibers of collagen to fill in and stitch together the injured area. Instead of merely replacing the strands that have been lost or severed, the skin forges a strong new bond with greater-than-normal amounts of collagen. Like the thread used to darn torn cloth, the new fibers are more numerous and closely gathered than the original strands. This collection of densely packed collagen threads is what is known as fibrotic tissue, or more popularly, "scar tissue."

While the body is constructing its fibrous bond of scar tissue, it simultaneously is rebuilding other parts of the skin structure, including stretchy strands of elastin, pigment-producing melanocytes, hair follicles, sweat and oil glands and nerves. It is aided in this by a process known as angiogenesis, in which a host of new blood vessels forms in the area to nourish all of the rapidly growing new tissues. The presence of these nutrient-supplying vessels makes the healing skin appear red on the surface. The color starts to fade once all of the new structures are formed. No longer needed to nourish rapidly growing cells, the auxiliary vessels gradually wither and disappear to be replaced with normal skin blood vessels.

The eventual shape, color and texture of the permanent scar that marks the once injured area is determined by how successful the skin has been in restoring all of its tiny parts despite the crowding presence of tightly packed collagen. Due to the presence of this fibrotic tissue, the scar will always be somewhat firm to the touch. Its surface will be smooth, perhaps even shiny, because scar tissue stretches and thins the epidermis like a balloon. To a greater or lesser degree, the scar will also be more pale in color than adjacent skin because there will be relatively fewer melanocytes in the area; and it will be less elastic, because it will contain fewer strands of elastin—the protein fibers that give skin its ability to stretch and snap back.

"BAD SCARS"

What people consider to be a "bad scar"—one that is very noticeable or disfiguring—forms when, for some reason, the skin cannot follow the normal blueprint for repair. This happens whenever a wound covers an area too large or deep for the skin to bridge normally. A bad burn, any exceptionally deep or extensive injury, and excisional surgery such as that performed to remove large skin tumors are all examples. Abnormally contoured or unusually red scars, which may form over a wound of any size or severity, occur when there is some glitch in the normal repair process. There can be any number of causes, including diseases or medical conditions that interfere with a person's individual wound healing mechanism. Some people simply heal poorly, for no reason that a doctor can pin down. Whatever the direct cause, the effect can be either a depressed (atrophic) scar or an abnormally raised (hypertrophic) scar.

ATROPHIC SCARS. Atrophic scarring occurs when new collagen does not grow back fully into a wound, although it may collect around the sides and beneath the injured area. The result is a depression lined in fibrotic scar tissue. The most familiar examples of atrophic scarring are the pits and pockmarks left by acne or chickenpox. But an atrophic scar can occur anywhere on the body after surgery or a deep injury.

Atrophic surgical or traumatic scars are treated with the same pulsed carbon dioxide laser that is used to resurface skin pitted by acne scars or lined with wrinkles (see Chapter 2). The laser vaporizes the scar and an area of surrounding skin, creating a new wound, broader and flatter than the atrophic depression; the new skin cells generated to heal the wound cover a more smoothly contoured area. The appearance of the scar is also improved by the laser's long-term effect on the skin's collagen-producing mechanism. As also happens after resurfacing with the CO_2 laser, collagen fibers in the laser-treated area grow back smoother and more regular in shape than before. In other words, more like normal collagen than like fibrous scar tissue. Although doctors do not understand the reasons why, an atrophic scar often continues to steadily improve, with further normalization in texture, for up to a year following laser treatment. The changes in appearance may be subtle, but they are clearly perceptible.

HYPERTROPHIC SCARS. Sometimes, a scar gets stuck in its early stage of development, when new collagen is rapidly growing. Fed by the auxiliary blood vessels that arise during healing, the collagen proliferates far beyond the point necessary to repair the wounded area. Pressed up by excess collagen, the resulting scar rises high above the surface of the skin. It is usually nodular in texture and colored an angry red from the excess blood vessels. This is known medically as a hypertrophic and erythematous scar. As well as being raised and red, it may also be chronically painful because the excess tissue presses on small nerves in the area. And it may itch because increased cellular activity releases substances that can stimulate prickling or tingling sensations.

TINA ALSTER, M.D. & LYDIA PRESTON

Raised red scars can occur anywhere on the body, although some parts are especially prone to developing them. They are most likely to occur over bony areas such as the mid-chest and thus are very common following open heart surgery, which has traditionally been performed through an eight-to-14-inch incision straight down the sternum. Raised red scars are also common on the skin overlying joints, occurring with special frequency over the shoulder or shoulder blade. Red hypertrophic scars are also common following mastectomy and breast augmentation or reduction surgery because skin on the breasts is relatively thin and delicate.

KELOIDS. Keloids are a more extreme version of hypertrophic scars. By definition, a keloid is a scar that grows beyond the boundaries of the original injury. The scar tissue behaves almost like a tumor because of its wild overgrowth of collagen. In appearance, a keloid is elevated and rounded with irregular clawlike margins. Its gristle-like texture is extremely hard to the touch. Under laboratory examination, the collagen strands that comprise a keloid look like dense balls of knotted string, interlaced with small blood vessels. Anyone can develop a keloid on any part of the body, although this type of scarring is more frequently found on darker skin types, particularly on people of African descent. Keloids are also somewhat more common on young women than on older women or men, suggesting to researchers that there may be a hormonal cause.

Together, hypertrophic and keloid scars affect upwards of 15 percent of the general population. As well as being slightly more common among people with darker skin types, they also frequently occur on individuals with medical disorders that affect their ability to produce collagen. People who get these hard raised scars usually say they started to feel them coming on about three weeks after the skin was injured—at about the time the scar from a wound that was healing normally would start to lighten and soften. "I knew something was wrong almost right away," said one woman, who developed a hypertrophic scar around her mouth following cosmetic surgery. "It felt wrong, stiff."

Doctors have a number of treatments for hypertrophic scars and keloids. One of the most frequently employed is direct injection of the scar with steroids, which reduce inflammation and, in effect, "stun" fibroblasts, the cells that produce collagen. The fibroblasts' output slows and the scar stops growing. However, steroids have several deleterious side effects. They can cause tissue atrophy, shrinking not only the scar itself but adjacent tissues as well. They also promote the formation of additional blood vessels. Scars injected with steroids thus frequently develop visible networks of spidery red vessels, or even large ropy veins.

Doctors sometimes try to treat unsightly raised scars by surgical excision, cutting out the fibrotic tissue and stitching up the resulting incision in the hope of creating a smaller, less obvious scar. Similarly, they occasionally attempt to reduce unsightly scars through dermabrasion. In recent years, doctors have also used the pulsed carbon dioxide resurfacing laser to vaporize raised scar tissue. Unfortunately, the very presence of a raised scar means that the affected patient is more than usually prone to hypertrophic scarring in that area. So any scar that has been removed—whether it has been cut out, subjected to dermabrasion or vaporized by a laser beam—is very likely to return, often worse than before.

Other treatments include freezing raised scars with liquid nitrogen, subjecting them to radiation and wrapping them with silicone gel sheeting, which through some unknown mechanism, promotes scar tissue shrinkage in some people. None of these methods has ever proven to be more than partially effective; most often scars either do not respond to treatment or they grow back afterwards.

LASER TREATMENT OF SCARS

Doctors now realize that the most effective laser for treating raised scars is not the CO_2 resurfacing laser that vaporizes the abnormal fibrotic tissue, but the 585nm flashlamp-pumped pulsed dye laser—the same vascular-specific laser that is used to treat port-wine birthmarks and other blood vessel anomalies. Physicians discovered this laser's effect on scars in the course of treating patients with port-wine stains. Individuals who happened to have scars on their birthmarked skin noticed that as the red color faded following laser therapy, the superimposed scars appeared to shrink and become more normal in surface texture than they had been before.

This observation inspired experiments on the laser's effect on other scars. One of the earliest controlled studies applied the 585nm pulsed dye laser to 16 patients with abnormally raised red scars from open heart surgery. The top half of each long, vertical scar was treated with the laser, the bottom half was left alone as a control. Each patient was treated twice, with laser sessions spaced six to eight weeks apart.

The results were dramatic. In every scar, the treated area almost immediately became softer, less red and considerably flatter. Before treatment, the height of the scars had ranged from 5 to 7 mm; after treatment, the average height was 2 mm. The treated scars felt more like normal skin to the touch. And every one of the patients who had suffered from persistent burning and itching reported that the pain and itchiness in the laser-irradiated halves of their scars disappeared after the first treatment. There were no changes at all in the untreated bottom halves of the scars. Long-term follow-up of the patients indicated that the beneficial changes were permanent.

There is no simple explanation to account for these exceptional improvements. Just as it does when removing birthmarks, the 585nm pulsed dye laser acts by destroying blood vessels, in this case, those present within the scar. It is easy to see how that takes out the scar's red color. It is harder to understand how the laser also debulks a scar so significantly or improves the way it feels to the patient.

Biopsies comparing laser-treated scar tissue with untreated scar tissue from the same patients show tremendous differences in the collagen structure. In the treated scars, the collagen fibers are measurably finer, softer and less densely packed than in untreated scars. No one has yet definitively identified the mechanism behind these changes, although a number of researchers are actively investigating the many possible biochemical factors at work.

In the meantime, the 585nm pulsed dye laser has proven itself repeatedly as an effective treatment for raised scars. Other controlled studies, as well as an increasing body of practical experience in doctors' offices, have shown the laser to affect striking improvements in many types of hypertrophic scars, including various surgical and traumatic scars and raised acne scars. Even raised scars that are white in color, and thus offer no obvious target for the vascular-specific laser's beam, will flatten out and assume a more normal texture following laser irradiation.

Doctors are also using the laser to treat scars left by other lasers, particularly the old, first-generation, continuous wave lasers that frequently burned patients. The argon laser once used on port-wine birthmarks often produced raised, nodular burn scars, stemming from heat build-up in the irradiated tissues. After successive treatments with the 585nm pulsed dye laser, these scars have shown appreciable changes, becoming increasingly lighter, flatter and taking on more of the surface characteristics of normal skin. More recently, doctors have used the 585nm pulsed dye laser to reduce the raised red scars that are a fortunately rare, but disastrous complication of overly aggressive laser resurfacing surgery with the new pulsed and scanned CO_2 lasers.

In most scar cases, two treatments with the 585nm pulsed dye laser produce significant improvement. Very hard, fibrous scars and keloids typically require more sessions—up to six or more. Patients with lighter skin tones (phototypes I-III) tend to respond more quickly to the laser; the scars in darker skin absorb less laser energy because the extra melanin filters the light.

The impact of the laser beam on the scar is said to feel like the snap of a rubber band. Most patients are treated without anesthesia; some people rub on a topical anesthetic 30 to 60 minutes before the procedure to numb the sting. A mild burning sensation, similar to a sunburn, usually follows treatment. Bluish purple bruises (purpura) mark the site of each laser pulse; these typically fade in seven to 10 days. The most common side effect is skin darkening (hyperpigmentation), caused by laser stimulation of the pigment producing cells in and around the scar. Left to its own, hyperpigmentation may take six months to a year to fade, provided the spots are not subjected to sun exposure. The fading can be speeded up by applying a topical bleaching cream containing hydroquinone or other melanin-inhibiting ingredients.

To allow time for adequate healing between laser exposures, treatments are spaced at six to eight week intervals, usually continuing until the treated scar shows no continued improvement. On scars that have become hyperpigmented, treatment is usually postponed until after the brown discoloration has cleared away.

BURN SCARS

Laser surgeons who treat burn victims use the same laser and basic laser procedure on the very extensive, usually raised, scars left by serious burns and the process of skin grafting that constitutes the first stage of burn care. Because large burns leave virtually no raw material to generate new skin cells over the affected areas, doctors compensate with skin grafts. Wherever possible, and particularly to cover highly visible areas such as the face, they employ what are known as full-thickness grafts—sheets of normal skin taken from inconspicuous locations and transplanted to the burned sections. Other areas are overlaid with partial thickness skin grafts, very thin strips of skin placed like latticework over the burns. These grafts do not replace the missing skin, but instead give the body substance to work with in producing new skin tissue. The cells in partial thickness grafts serve as mother cells which, in effect, "seed" the growth of new collagen and epidermal tissue.

Both types of graft leave troublesome scars. Full thickness grafts are commonly circumscribed by a thin, hard line of scar tissue to mark the border between the transplanted skin and its surroundings. Partial thickness grafts produce thick, ropy scars that not only are terribly disfiguring, but can also be crippling. As the scars develop and harden, the fibrous tissue in them contracts as if stiffening into protective stasis. Elizabeth said that as the grafts on her arms, chest, back and upper thighs healed, the cord-like scars pulled at her like a puppeteer's strings. They drew her fingers into claws, flexed her limbs into rigid immobility, and twisted her torso forward into a distorted fetal position. This was the shape her body had assumed when, after nearly three months of acute hospital care, she entered an inpatient rehabilitation facility.

Over the following months, she underwent intensive physical therapy to counteract the scar contraction. For seven hours a day therapists pulled and stretched her limbs and manipulated her scar-covered joints to give her the mobility she needed to stand, walk and perform ordinary daily tasks, such as eating or brushing her teeth. But even a few days respite from this intensive regimen, and her scars would start to draw back in. Those on her torso, she said, "felt like an iron cage." This was when she became so depressed by her plight that she seriously contemplated suicide.

But at about the same time, Elizabeth learned about work being done on burn scars by a few dermatological laser specialists. Although one of the plastic surgeons who was working on her case warned her that laser surgery on scars such as hers was "not proved," and would probably be a waste of time and effort, she decide to try laser therapy.

Within 24 hours after the first of what would be a series of treatments with the 585nm pulsed dye laser, Elizabeth noticed welcome changes. The red, ridged surgical scars surrounding the skin graft that had been applied to her face like a mask, softened and blanched. Those on her torso and limbs became more pliable. The second treatment further reduced the negative grip of the scars on her body. "Whatever living force was in them, the laser took out," she marveled, demonstrating the ease with which she could extend her fingers and raise and lower her arms. Although a long road toward recovery still lay ahead, Elizabeth stopped thinking about ending her life and began considering how she could rebuild it.

In terms of serious effects, stretch marks lie at the opposite end of the spectrum from terrible burn scars such as Elizabeth's. These thin, shiny, slightly indented and wrinkled lines that appear on the body after the skin has been stretched beyond its capacity to snap back, are in no way harmful or genuinely disfiguring. But most people who acquire them view them as unsightly, and they fervently wish to be rid of them. Unfortunately, not even lasers can erase stretch marks, although one day they may prove able to do so. In the meantime, they have demonstrated some ability to provide modest improvements in the marks on some people.

Although patients regard them as scars, stretch marks, medically known as striae distensae, technically speaking are not scars, because they are not comprised of fibrotic tissue. Instead they represent an absence of tissue—gaps in the dermis left by stretched or torn elastin fibers just beneath the skin's surface. They occur following rapid gains in body size that abruptly stretch the skin. Striae first appear as deep red marks that gradually fade to a silvery white color. The epidermis over the mark thins out somewhat, giving the surface a fragile feel and appearance.

Adolescents frequently acquire stretch marks during growth spurts, commonly on the breasts, hips, buttocks or thighs. Up to 50 percent of all women develop them on the abdomen or breasts during pregnancy. Body builders often get stretch marks over areas of large muscle mass. The tendency to develop stretch marks appears to be inherited; it may be exacerbated by the hormonal changes of pregnancy, or the use of birth control pills or systemic steroids.

Many commercial creams and lotions purport either to

prevent stretch marks by softening and supposedly increasing the flexibility of skin, or to lessen the appearance of marks that already exist. None of these remedies penetrate deeply enough into the skin to reach the dermis where the affected elastin fibers lie. Even if they could get through to the dermis, the ingredients in commercial creams have no medical effect on dermal tissues. So far, the only proved treatment for striae is the topical anti-acne medication, Retin-A. Applied to new, still-red stretch marks, high concentrations of Retin-A seem to stimulate the growth of new dermal blood vessels and promote collagen and elastin repair. On some people, this appears to help knit the torn dermis back together, thus eliminating the mark—or at least making it less noticeable than it would otherwise be.

In recent years, the collagen-modulating effect of the 585nm pulsed dye laser on raised scars has inspired doctors to experimentally use the same laser on stretch marks. The results have been mixed and generally disappointing to patients. Stretch marks are treated in the same fashion as scars, with a series of laser pulses that leave a line of faint purple purpura down the length of each mark. As this bruising fades, the marks usually retain some color, a mild inflammation that makes red marks darker, and white marks pinkish or somewhat lavender-colored. This coloring takes a few weeks to fade. During that time, some patients report that the treated areas seem to fill in somewhat and take on a surface texture more like that of normal skin. As with Retin-A treatment, red, recently acquired stretch marks seem to improve more markedly than older, white marks.

Computer analysis of skin surface replicas (rubberized impressions) taken of laser-treated stretch marks confirm these subjective impressions. Stretch marks are indeed somewhat smoother after laser treatment than untreated ones, with recent red marks showing the most significant improvement. Moreover, some researchers have detected increased elastic and collagen fibers in biopsies of laser-irradiated stretch marks. So obviously the laser beam has a real effect.

The question for patients remains, is there enough of an effect to make laser treatment worthwhile? One woman, treated for four-year-old post-pregnancy stretch marks on her abdomen, supplied an answer. "It's really up to the individual. I think mine got better and I'm glad I did it. But maybe that's just wishful thinking. My husband says he can't see the difference and why did I bother."

The final answer may come only after many more years of experimentation and technological development. Laser treatment of scars and scar-like stretch marks is a genuine medical frontier. The advances that have been made so far hold exciting and promising hope for the future.

SKIN CARE AFTER LASER TREATMENT FOR SCARS

The treated scars will be covered with blue-grey purpura (bruises) for up to ten days and must be treated with extreme care.

1. Apply bacitracin or polysporin ointment (not Neosporin, which causes allergic reactions in some people) to the bruised areas once or twice a day until they have faded. If the skin blisters or breaks, you may cover it with a nonstick bandage (Telfa pad with adhesive).

2. Take acetaminophen (such as Tylenol) to relieve any discomfort or pain; if pain persists past 24 hours, notify your doctor.

3. Avoid aspirin or any aspirin-containing medicines during the healing period (one to two weeks, or until the bruising has completely disappeared).

4. You may shower or bathe, but do not rub the scars with a washcloth. Pat them gently dry with a towel. The skin is extremely delicate after treatment and it can easily be broken with vigorous rubbing.

5. To relieve any swelling, apply a gel ice pack—or a bag of frozen peas or corn—wrapped in a soft cloth, every hour for 10 to 15 minutes at a time.

6. Protect treated areas from sun exposure which can lead to permanent changes in pigmentation. Use a broad spectrum sunscreen with SPF 15 or higher throughout your course of treatment.

7. Avoid contact sports and do not go swimming while the area is healing (as long as the purpura are present).

CHAPTER TEN

THE LASER AS RAZOR:
REMOVING UNWANTED HAIR

*F*or most women—and a good many men—it sounds like a dream come true. No more shaving, tweezing, plucking, waxing. Instead, farewell forever to unwanted hair, vaporized in a flash of laser light. And theoretically at least, the notion of using a laser to permanently depilate underarms, defuzz legs or strip the hair from a furry back is as feasible as using a laser to zero in on any other organic target, such as the abnormal blood vessels in a port-wine stain or the melanin-laden cells that make up an age spot. Technology does not quite measure up to theory, however. Permanent hair removal via the laser's beam has proved to be a goal just tantalizingly beyond reach.

Laser hair removal is, in essence, a high-tech version of electrolysis, which until now was the only way to permanently remove hair. In electrolysis, a fine needle is inserted into the hair follicle. An electric current is sent down the shaft, destroying the root of the hair and disabling the follicle's hair-producing mechanism. If all goes as intended, no hair will ever grow from that follicle again. Whether or not this actually occurs is always an open question. Electrolysis is exasperatingly unpredictable. It takes an experienced, highly skilled operator to place the needle precisely in order to deliver the electric current to just the right spot in the follicle. If the operator misses, the hair will grow back. It may grow back anyway, because the hair-producing root can only be destroyed at certain specific stages in the hair's complex, imperfectly understood growing cycle. And sometimes, not even perfect technique and timing combined spell success. Veteran electrolysis operators usually tell clients that as much as 30 percent of the hair in any given location will eventually grow back, no matter what.

Other problems with electrolysis abound. It is a tediously long and uncomfortable (yes, painful) process, taking many repeat treatments to defoliate any section of skin. Even an experienced operator can usually only treat a couple of hundred hairs in an hour. That usually covers only a few square inches—an average upper lip or one underarm. Sometimes the needle leaves small, fibrous scars. Other times, it damages the skin's pigment-producing cells, causing a loss or gain in skin color (hypopigmentation or hyperpigmentation). In those cases, dozens of permanent tiny white or brown spots may eventually mark where the electrolysis needle has been.

A number of laser companies have worked on developing technology that would send laser light rather than an electric current down the hair shaft to destroy hair at its root. The first to obtain Food and Drug Administration approval for their laser hair removal process was a company called ThermoLase, the subsidiary of a defense contractor better known as a manufacturer of high-tech devices that detect bombs and drugs.

Called SoftLight, this system is a proprietary technology supplied to physicians though special licensing arrangements.

Experience in the company-owned spas where it was first tested on humans, combined with the limited observations of the few doctors who have used it in their practices during its first year of availability, indicated that this laser system is similar to or even better than electrolysis in terms of long-term effectiveness. Like electrolysis, the SoftLight laser requires multiple treatments to remove what is described as a "cosmetically acceptable" percentage of the hair from any given location. ("Cosmetically acceptable" essentially means that the hair has been thinned out so much that only a relative handful of stray and inconspicuous hairs remain.) The laser's advantages over electrolysis are that it is far quicker and easier to use, it is non-invasive (no needles!), slightly less painful and it is less likely to produce scarring or other adverse side effects.

At this writing (mid-1996), SoftLight was the only laser hair removal device to have won FDA approval, and thus was the system with the most extensive available information on its performance. Other competing hair-removing lasers under FDA review at the time (i.e., Palomar Epilase) would be expected to produce similar results.

LASER HAIR REMOVAL

The SoftLight hair-removal laser is a modified, much less powerful version of the Nd:YAG laser used to remove tattoo pigment and brown spots. In this case, the laser's ultimate target is a small structure at the base of the hair follicle called the papilla, which nourishes the growth of new hair. The laser beam is absorbed by a sooty black solution that is applied to the skin beforehand and firmly rubbed in so that it goes all the way down into the hair follicle to the papilla. As the light from the laser beam is absorbed by the black pigment, heat travels straight down the shaft to the base to scorch the papilla. The heat actually generates a chemical reaction capable of killing this feeder structure.

The targeted area is usually waxed to remove all the hair immediately before laser treatment. (Patients are asked not to shave for at least five days beforehand.) This empties the follicles, leaving them open to take in the black conducting medium, an oily solution consisting largely of carbon in a mineral oil base. The operator aims the laser at the blackened areas of skin and immediately there is a crackling, rapid-fire popping sound. Large bright sparks, which result from the laser hitting the carbon in the conducting lotion, fly up like glittering spray from a Fourth of July sparkler. Any hairs that have not been removed by the waxing blanch as the beam strikes them; the heat destroys the melanin that gives them their color. Those hairs usually fall out within a couple of weeks.

The pain is minimal—less than any of the dermatologic lasers used to treat medical conditions. However, the steady barrage of laser pulses, and the heat they generate, can build to very uncomfortable levels. It may actually start to hurt if the laser-treated skin is in a sensitive anatomical site where there are more-than-average numbers of nerve endings, such as at the bikini line or at the base of the spine. "It does hurt, but it's not as bad as the waxing," commented one woman while having her upper lip lased. A man undergoing laser hair removal over his back described the sensation as "like needles falling on my skin." Others asked to evaluate the pain have described it as a tingling sensation or "like hot pin pricks."

Whatever the individual feels while the laser is being applied, the sensation ceases the instant the beam is turned off.

Immediately following treatment, the skin may turn pink; if this occurs, the color usually fades within hours. Very rarely, there may be some pinpoint bleeding from a hair follicle or two. This is probably due more to the waxing process than to the lasing. Otherwise, no complications from this form of laser treatment have been observed.

One very serious potential repercussion has arisen however—the dangerous threat the laser beam poses to unprotected eyes. Everyone in any room where a laser is being operated must wear protective safety goggles the entire time the laser is in use. The goggles are specifically designed to block the beams generated by specific lasers. A stray laser beam that inadvertently shines into an unprotected or improperly protected eye can instantly destroy the vision in that eye, and all medical personnel who work with lasers know that to remove their safety goggles while a laser is in use is to court disaster. But for some reason—perhaps because hair removal is not a medical procedure and it is usually performed in a spa-like atmosphere—this basic, critical precaution is sometimes violated when it comes to the hair removal laser. There have been a number of reported instances when clients and even some operators, who should know better, have pulled off their goggles while the laser was on, just to take a peek "and see how things are going." Although none of those safety violations resulted in injury, any one could have been calamitous. Always remember, if you are being treated with a laser, NEVER remove the goggles until the laser is switched off.

How It Works

So far, there is no consistently reliable permanent hair removal system of any kind. Like so much about the skin, the process by which hair grows is imperfectly understood. What is known is that human hair grows in cycles, each cycle comprised of three phases. In the anagen, or growing phase, the hair is actively increasing in length. In the telogen, or resting stage, the strand simply sits at its destined length for a period of time until it slips free of the follicle and falls out (the catagen phase). The same follicle then produces a successor hair.

At any one time, roughly 85 percent of any individual's hair follicles are actively nourishing and growing hairs; about 11 percent are holding on to resting hairs, and four percent are shedding hairs. These percentages may vary depending on the location of the hairs on the body. Similarly, the amount of time a hair remains in any one of the three phases of the growth cycle also depends in part on its location. The cycle is further affected to a greater or lesser degree by a number of biological factors, including hormones, drugs, stress, age, even body weight.

In order to successfully shut down the production of an individual hair, heat from the electrolysis needle or the laser beam must strike the hair's root during the active, anagen stage. At that time, the hair's growth is being sustained by blood vessels in the tiny bulb-like papilla, which lies at the base of the follicle. In both the resting and shedding phases of the cycle, the papilla atrophies or shrinks and thus easily escapes injury from any potentially destructive agent. But if the papilla is badly injured or destroyed during its active stage, it will never again nourish the growth of another hair. This is the goal in permanent hair removal. Unfortunately for anyone attempting to achieve that goal, the papillae are remarkably resilient. Even badly injured papillae demonstrate extraordinary ability to repair themselves and go on to produce new hair.

Receiving laser-assisted hair removal treatment does not guarantee total depilation. But different areas on different people respond in entirely different and unexpected ways. So the number of treatments required to obtain a cosmetically acceptable result on any given body part varies with each individual. While it is impossible to predict exactly how a particular person will respond, clinical experience so far indicates that the areas listed below generally seem to respond in the manner described.

UPPER LIP. This is a stubborn area, but minimally painful to treat. It usually takes three or more treatments, at four to eight week time intervals, to remove a cosmetically significant number of more than 500 hairs per square centimeter on the upper lip.

CHIN. The skin below the mouth is, if anything, even harder to treat than the skin above it, whether the patient is a man wishing to eliminate or thin his facial stubble, or a woman with a few stray bristles. Chin hair grows according to an extremely unpredictable growth cycle, so it is impossible to judge just when treatment will be most effective.

UNDERARMS. Underarm hair is very difficult to remove, requiring three or more treatments spaced six to eight weeks apart. Moreover, the pre-laser waxing is very painful, although the laser itself feels relatively innocuous to most people.

BIKINI LINE. The coarse hairs of the upper thigh at the bikini line have so far proved on the whole to be the most responsive of any to laser hair removal treatment. It tends to be painful, although less so than waxing. Three or more treatments, spaced from 1 to 2 months apart, have in many cases completely removed the hair, with no signs of it returning after a year or more on some people.

CHAPTER ELEVEN

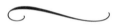

ON THE COSMETIC LASER HORIZON

*D*ermatologists compare the emergence of cosmetic lasers in the mid-1990s to the explosive proliferation of personal computers that began more than a decade earlier. In both cases a highly complex and sophisticated technology, previously available only to a small handful of skilled experts, developed to the point where seemingly overnight it became accessible to a wide population of new users. Cosmetic lasers are now working as dramatic a transformation on the practice of dermatology as did computers on the life of modern society as a whole.

Like computer science, laser technology is evolving rapidly, repeatedly relegating devices that had been considered state-of-the-art into early obsolescence. Lasers are becoming smaller, more versatile and easier to use. Some early dermatologic lasers are already as out of date as hand-cranked desktop adding machines. As was also the case with computers, lasers are becoming less expensive, quickening their spread into doctors' offices. This coupling of fast-improving technology with broadening availability almost ensures the development of new uses for cosmetic lasers.

Clinical experience in recent years has given doctors a wealth of knowledge about laser light's often unique effects on human tissue. This new understanding enables practitioners to manipulate existing lasers in unforeseen ways, designing innovative therapies that make the most of the laser's power while minimizing damaging side effects. Along with this information about the laser's impact on living cells has come important new insights into basic biologic processes: how wounds heal, how blood vessels in the skin function, how our hair grows, what gives our complexions their color, the myriad ways our skin changes as we age. Most of the laser procedures described in this book are regarded as first generation versions of more advanced therapies that doctors expect to employ in the future as they learn how to better "program" their machines to do many more things.

The following are some of the areas under active investigation:

EXPECTED REFINEMENTS IN EXISTING LASER PROCEDURES

▶ ENHANCED RESURFACING TECHNIQUES. As doctors learn more about how the collagen and elastin fibers that make up the skin's basic scaffolding respond to laser impact, they expect to become even more successful at smoothing away wrinkles and the indented scars caused by acne.

▶ TREATING VASCULAR MALFORMATIONS. The 585nm flash-lamp-pumped pulse dye laser now widely used on various skin disorders was invented to treat the small shallow vessels that cause children's port-wine stains, hair's-width vessels lying .5 to 1 mm beneath the skin surface. But many vascular skin disorders involve larger vessels situated deeper below the surface. Doctors have recently begun using lasers that can be adjusted more precisely, enabling them to zero in on such targets as leg veins, large mixed hemangiomas and the thickened components of adult port-wine stains.

▶ REFINEMENTS IN SCAR IMPROVEMENT TECHNIQUES, INCLUDING REMOVAL OF STRETCH MARKS. The serendipitous discovery of the 585nm pulsed dye laser's ability to improve the appearance of many types of scars only suggests that more precisely tuning it to those specific targets would result in even more effective therapy. Moreover, as doctors learn more about scar formation, they expect to discover ways to intervene in the scar forming process, timing laser treatments to prevent disfiguring scars from ever forming in the first place.

▶ MORE EFFICIENT MEANS OF REMOVING TATTOOS AND BROWN SPOTS. Laser surgeons still do not understand precisely how their machines work to eradicate the pigments in tattoo inks or the natural pigment melanin in brown lesions such as age spots, moles, freckles, melasma and other patchy brown marks. Nor do they understand why some patients seem to respond more efficiently than others to laser therapy for these lesions. As physicians study laser impact on these complex little entities embedded in the skin, they expect to come up with ways to adjust laser light so that fewer, less painful and more precise treatments will be needed to remove any sort of pigmented mark.

TINA ALSTER, M.D. & LYDIA PRESTON

► **REMOVING UNWANTED HAIR.** Learning how to better predict and track hair-growing cycles on different parts of the body should allow physicians to be more precise in disabling hair follicles and permanently removing unwanted hair.

NEW LASER TARGETS

► **UNDER-EYE CIRCLES.** Resurfacing around the eyes with the high-energy pulsed carbon dioxide laser can have a dramatic effect on dark under-eye circles, minimizing their appearance in the smoother, tighter skin. But very sooty-looking "raccoon eyes" are due to the presence of excess skin pigment that may be unaffected by the CO_2 laser. Some experiments using pigment-specific lasers such as those more commonly employed on tattoos or brown lesions have shown promise in reducing excess pigment around the eyes and thus the appearance of dark circles.

► **PSORIASIS.** A chronic skin disease, psoriasis is characterized by clearly delineated red patches overlaid with white scales. These lesions, for which there is no known cause, come from the growth of excess blood vessels, coupled with overproduction of superficial skin cells. There is no cure for psoriasis, but some physicians have had limited success in reducing individual lesions by treating the proliferating small blood vessels with the same vascular-specific lasers used on other vascular malformations.

► **OIL GLANDS AND SWEAT GLANDS.** Just as doctors are learning how to use lasers to shut down the live hair-nourishing papilla at the base of the hair follicle, they are also investigating ways to target and disable sweat glands and oil-producing sebaceous glands. Slowing the production of oil or sweat on some areas of the body could conceivably make acne breakouts, an overly shiny nose or chronically damp underarms things of the past.

PHOTODYNAMIC LASER THERAPY

One of the first jobs scientists ever envisioned for medical lasers employed a technique called photodynamic therapy (PDT)—sometimes known as photochemotherapy or photoradiation therapy. Principally designed as a treatment for cancerous tumors, PDT involves injecting a special photosensitizing substance into an area where it is selectively absorbed by the malignant cells. The tumor is then irradiated with a laser (or other light source) which converts the drug into a toxic substance that in turn kills the cancerous cells.

Use of this promising method of precisely targeting and eliminating cancerous tissue has been severely limited, in part because of serious side effects associated with the various photosensitizing substances. So far, PDT has been approved in only a few countries for use on patients with certain types of internal cancers. (The therapeutic light is delivered to the site within the body by means of a flexible fiberoptic cable.)

The use of PDT in dermatology remains very much an investigational therapy, currently being studied in a handful of research centers. However, physicians still feel that it holds promise as a treatment for skin cancer, including basal and squamous cell cancers, melanoma and Kaposi's sarcoma. It may also prove useful in the future for noncancerous skin conditions such as psoriasis, viral infections, hair removal and some types of vascular malformations.

LASER-ASSISTED PLASTIC SURGERY

One of the most exciting new uses for lasers is as adjunct surgical tools in conventional cosmetic surgery. Plastic surgeons have long been attracted to the tightly focused laser beam as a cutting tool because it cauterizes small blood vessels as it goes, making clean, bloodless incisions in areas such as the face or scalp that are especially prone to bleeding. Today, the same technological advances that have given dermatologists increased control over lasers have opened new opportunities for cosmetic surgeons. Cosmetic surgical procedures in which lasers can contribute to improved results include:

▶ **EYELIFTS:** Lasers make clean precise incisions in the delicate eyelid and brow areas and lead to reduced bleeding in the operative field.

▶ **FULL FACE LIFTS:** Lasers not only make incisions, but also can evaporate small pockets of fat.

▶ **LIPOSUCTION:** Lasers can help to cut and free skin from underlying tissue before subcutaneous fat is vacuumed out.

▶ **HAIR TRANSPLANTS:** Lasers can make small incisions in which to plant the new hair. Doctors experimenting with laser-assisted hair transplant surgery are learning that in many cases, the hair plugs are less likely to be rejected, the scalp heals faster, the hair begins to grow more quickly, and the appearance is more natural than with conventional techniques.

Generally, laser-assisted plastic surgery can lead to quicker recovery and less postoperative swelling and pain than operations performed solely with the scalpel and other traditional surgical tools. And surgeons who are very experienced in laser techniques can substantially reduce the time involved in a procedure, thus lessening risk and discomfort for the patient.

APPENDIX A

THE RIGHT LASER FOR THE JOB

$\mathcal{T}$he cosmetic lasers likely to be found in a dermatologist's or plastic surgeon's office today fall into two broad categories: pulsed and continuous wave. On the whole, by far the safest and most effective lasers for the skin are the newer pulsed or scanned lasers. At the present time, continuous wave lasers are regarded as having only limited use in dermatology. They have a somewhat broader range of applications in cosmetic surgery, where they are sometimes employed as incisional tools. Here is a summary of the most common of the currently available machines in both categories:

PULSED LASERS

HIGH-ENERGY PULSED OR SCANNED CARBON DIOXIDE LASER (Examples: Coherent UltraPulse, Sharplan Silktouch, Tissue Technologies TruPulse, Luxar NovaPulse)

Used for: Resurfacing skin to remove wrinkles, depressed (atrophic) acne scars and other depressed scars from surgery or trauma. Extensive sun damage, pre-cancerous growths (actinic chelitis, actinic keratoses) and some basal cell cancers. Also to vaporize superficial skin growths (skin tags, seborrheic keratoses, dermatosis papulosa nigra, linear epidermal nevi). Benign dermal tumors (including angiofibromas, neurofibromas, sebaceous hyperplasia, rhinophyma, syringomas, xanthelasma). The scaly, superficial portion of some warts. Flesh-colored, raised moles (benign compound nevi) .

Q-SWITCHED ALEXANDRITE

Used for: Tattoo removal (especially for black, blue-black and green pigments); pigmented dermal or combination lesions such as blue nevus, nevus of Ota, nevus of Ito and benign moles.

Q-SWITCHED NEODYNIUM: YTTRIUM-ALUMINUM-GARNET (ND: YAG)

This laser can be adjusted to emit two different wave-lengths, depending on the application it is being used for.

ND: YAG (1064 NM)

Used for: Tattoo removal (especially for black and blue-black pigments); deep dermal pigmented lesions (blue nevus, nevus of Ota, nevus of Ito). In a patented process, utilizing a carbon-based solution to remove or thin hair in selected locations.

Nd: YAG (532 nm)

Used for: Tattoo removal (red, orange and yellow pigments). Superficial brown pigmented lesions (café-au-lait birthmarks, freckles, age spots, some brown moles)

Q-Switched Ruby

Used for: Tattoo removal (black, blue-black and green pigments.) Superficial and deep pigmented lesions (i.e. freckles, age spots and café-au-lait birthmarks; post-inflammatory hyperpigmentation), nevus of Ota, benign moles.

Flashlamp-Pumped Pulsed Dye

Currently, there are two versions of this laser in common use, each utilizing a different nanometer (nm) wavelength:

585nm

Used for: Red birthmarks, i.e. port-wine stains and hemangiomas. Dilated capillaries (telangiectasias) and chronic redness (erythema) associated with rosacea, sun damage and other causes. Superficial red growths (cherry angiomas, spider angiomas, venous lakes, pyogenic granulomas). The feeder vessels of some warts and the vascular component of some benign dermal tumors (ie., angofibromas). Also used in scar revision, especially for raised (hypertrophic) red scars (i.e. burn, surgical or acne scars), keloids, and stretch marks.

510NM PIGMENTED LESION DYE LASER (PLDL)

Used for: Epidermal pigmented lesions such as café-au-lait birthmarks, freckles, age spots. Some brown moles (ie., junctional nevi). Tattoo removal (red, orange and yellow pigments).

CONTINUOUS WAVE LASERS

CONTINUOUS WAVE CARBON DIOXIDE

Used for: Some plastic surgery incisions, eyelid operations, some forms of nail surgery. Occasionally to vaporize superficial growths, although its application for this use is limited because of the danger of scarring from heat build-up.

ARGON LASER AND ARGON-PUMPED TUNABLE DYE

Used for: Removing large resistant vessels in hemangiomas or nodules in advanced port-wine stains. Sometimes for large telangiectasias.

KTP, COPPER BROMIDE, KRYPTON AND COPPER VAPOR

Used for: Small vascular lesions (ie., cherry angiomas) or large telangiectasias.

APPENDIX B

WHAT LASER SURGERY COSTS
AND HOW TO PAY FOR IT

*B*elow is a list of ballpark figures for the various treatments discussed in the book along with some anecdotally-based impressions of the odds you might encounter in getting insurance reimbursement. Bear in mind that the prices you find may vary substantially according to individual physicians' policies. Also, most laser surgeons set individual prices based on how extensive an area of skin is involved. Prices given here are per treatment; remember that many skin conditions require multiple laser sessions.

LASER RESURFACING

*(For wrinkles or acne scarring, Chapters 1-3,
or extensive sun damage, Chapter 4)*

Costs should include anesthesia and a specified number of follow-up visits for at least the first post-operative month. Pre- or post-operative medications generally are not included in these fees.

Full Face: $2,500-$8,000

Around the Eyes: $800-$2,000

Around the mouth: $800-$2,500 (Higher figures generally represent a larger cosmetic unit, i.e., the area around the mouth plus the nasolabial folds and/or the chin.)

Upper Lip Only: $400-$750

Cheeks (usually for acne scarring): $1,000-$2,800

Chances for insurance reimbursement: Virtually none for wrinkles or sun damage; sometimes companies will pay part of the costs for acne scarring. Fair chance of reimbursement for treatment undertaken for precancerous growths, although most companies will pay only what they consider to be their usual and customary fees for any form of treatment (always lower in price than typical laser fees).

Skin Growths

(Chapter 4)

Superficial Epidermal or Dermal Lesions: $150-$1,000 depending on size of the area or the number of lesions.

Warts: $150-$600

Skin cancers and pre-cancers: $150-1,000 for isolated or scattered lesions depending on size and number; up to $8,000 (full-face resurfacing for extensive sun-damage).

Lip resurfacing for actinic chelitis: $500-$1,500

Nose resurfacing (for rhinophyma): $500-$1,500

Chances for insurance reimbursement: Very poor except for cancers and some precancers. Most insurance companies regard benign skin tumors as cosmetic conditions, unless they are located in an area where they cause pain or interfere with a vital function such as eyesight. In those cases, and for cancers or precancers, companies may pay—although often only what they consider to be their usual and customary fees for other therapy for the same condition.

BROWN LESIONS

(Chapter 5)

AGE SPOTS AND FRECKLES, DERMAL LESIONS, HYPERPIGMENTATION: $200-$1,000
MOLES: $350-$1,000
CAFÉ-AU-LAIT SPOTS: $350-$1,000

Chances for insurance reimbursement: Very poor except for abnormal (precancerous) moles or café-au-lait birthmarks on children.

TATTOO REMOVAL

(Chapter 6)

PROFESSIONAL, COSMETIC OR TRAUMATIC: $200-$1,000

Chances for insurance reimbursement: Very rare for professional or cosmetic tattoos; fair chance for traumatic tattoos.

RED BIRTHMARKS

(Chapter 7)

PORT-WINE STAINS: Typically $350-$600 per treatment, for a moderate-sized mark; $1,000-$2,000 for an extensive area such as the whole face or an entire limb.
HEMANGIOMAS: $250-$600 per treatment.

Chances for insurance reimbursement: Usually good for children with port-wine stains; very poor for children with hemangiomas because most companies regard them as a condition that will clear up without treatment (even though many hemangiomas cause significant damage, such as impinging on an eye and threatening sight). Most companies are reluctant to reimburse expenses for treatment of adult port-wine stains, even large invasive ones, apparently acting on the theory that adults have adjusted to their birthmarks and therefore no longer regard them as disfiguring—a premise that any adult with a port-wine stain knows from bitter experience is untrue.

OTHER RED BLEMISHES

(Chapter 8)

VISIBLE VEINS (TELANGIECTASIAS): $150-$800 depending on number of veins and size of area.
ROSACEA: $150-$800 depending on size of area.
POIKILODERMA: $400-$1,200, depending on size of area.
CHERRY ANGIOMAS AND OTHER SMALL VASCULAR GROWTHS: $150-$800, depending on the number treated.

Chances for insurance reimbursement: Poor in general, although often good for rosacea patients who suffer from persistent discomfort associated with flushing episodes. Chances are variable for cherry angiomas and pyogenic granulomas, which some companies regard as tumors. Poikiloderma may or may not be covered.

SCARS

(Chapter 9)

DEPRESSED (ATROPHIC) SCARS: Same as for resurfacing, roughly $350 up to several thousand depending on the size of the area.

RAISED (HYPERTROPHIC) RED SCARS AND KELOIDS: $250 - $1,000

BURNS: $250 - $2,000 and up depending on size.

STRETCH MARKS: $250-$650, depending on size, number and location.

Chances for insurance reimbursement: Good for burns, traumatic and surgical scars, especially if they cause pain or discomfort from itching or burning. However, many companies will only pay their usual and customary fees, which may not cover typical laser costs. Poor chance of reimbursement for stretch marks and acne scars.

HAIR REMOVAL

(Chapter 10)

Fees below are typical for a single initial laser hair removal session. Because multiple treatments are usually needed, there may be a percentage reduction for subsequent sessions.

UPPER LIP: $500
CHIN: $750
UNDERARMS: $600
BACK: $600
BIKINI LINE: $600
LOWER LEGS: $900
UPPER LEGS: $900

Chances for insurance reimbursement: May have a chance if hair growth is related to medical conditions that cause hirsutism. This treatment is so new that most insurance companies will regard it as experimental, if not purely cosmetic.

APPENDIX C

CHOOSING A LASER SPECIALIST

*A*s when selecting any doctor, you must carefully shop around when looking for a qualified cosmetic laser specialist. Your task may be made difficult by the fact that dermatologic laser surgery is a new and rapidly evolving specialty. For this reason, there are relatively few practitioners with extensive experience in the field.

Start by asking your own physician to recommend a laser specialist. You may also contact the American Society for Dermatologic Surgery at 930 North Meacham Road, Schaumburg, IL 60173 (telephone 1-800-441-2737). Ask for the names of board-certified dermatologists in your area who include laser surgery as a specialty. Or write to the American Society for Laser Medicine and Surgery at 2404 Stewart Square, Wausau, WI 54401 for the names of members in your area. Be aware, however, that any physician can join this latter society simply by filling out an application and paying annual dues. So membership does not guarantee special competence,

---

although it is indicative of interest in keeping up with developments in the field.

For any laser procedure, you'll want to be assured ahead of time that the doctor knows what he or she is doing. For a major procedure that may cost you considerable pain, time and money, such as full-face resurfacing, you will wish to make every effort to find the very best person for the job. In that case, try to come up with three doctors to interview and then make appointments for consultations with each. Here are some questions you can take along:

1. **How did you become interested in laser surgery and what kind of training did you receive?**

   The answers here should give you some idea of how interested the doctor is in lasers and how long that interest has been nurtured. In terms of training, look for academic courses (which have in recent years become a mandatory part of training in dermatology) or some period of time observing and practicing under the wing of a more experienced laser specialist. Training courses offered by laser companies offer only minimal preparation.

2. **Do you rent or own your own lasers?**

   To keep costs down, some doctors periodically rent a specific laser for a day or two and schedule a number of appropriate procedures for those days. For the most part, this is a dead giveaway that the doctor lacks clinical experience with that laser and the procedures it performs. However, to be fair, sometimes very well-trained young physicians just starting out may have no other choice than to rent costly lasers.

3. **How many procedures have you performed for this condition?**

You want to find a doctor who has particular interest—and adequate experience—in your condition.

4. **Can I see before and after photographs of patients you have treated?**

Like other cosmetic practitioners, cosmetic laser specialists document their procedures carefully with photographs. Physicians with extensive experience should be able to show you samples of their work. Be sure you insist on seeing pictures of that doctor's own patients. Doctors who do not have a large backlog of patients will sometimes try to show you photographs obtained from laser companies—or from other more experienced doctors.

5. **May I talk to one or two of your patients who have had the same procedure?**

Although many doctors make it a policy not to give out the names of patients under any circumstance, some will put you in touch with those who have volunteered to give a reference. It's worth asking.

6. **Have you published any articles on laser surgery in peer-reviewed journals? Have you lectured to other doctors on the subject?**

In a new specialty such as laser surgery, the most active practitioners commonly share their experiences by publishing articles and speaking before their colleagues. A doctor that has done this is likely to have more interest and competence in the field, and also probably keeps well abreast of current findings and developments.

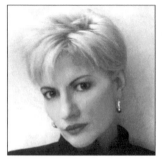

Tina Alster, M.D., is internationally recognized as one of the leading practitioners of cosmetic laser surgery. She has directed pioneering research projects that have contributed to the development of today's most widely used cosmetic lasers. She is also the author of numerous medical papers and two authoritative textbooks on the subject of laser surgery. In private practice since 1990, as founding director of The Washington Institute of Dermatologic Laser Surgery, Dr. Alster is on the Medical faculties at Georgetown and Harvard Universities. She lives in Washington, DC with her husband and infant son.

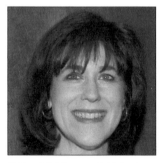

Lydia Preston, a long-time writer and editor at Time-Life Books, worked on many of the company's most successful and innovative popular series, including "Home Repair and Improvement," "The Old West," "The Seafarers," "World War II," "Understanding Computers," "Your Health," "Mysteries of the Unknown," and "The American Indians." She has written consumer and health-related features for *Money Magazine*, *National Geographic Traveler* and *The Washington Post Magazine*. She lives in Alexandria, Virginia, with her husband and two young sons.